Do you feel like you're 80 years old, and you're only 40 or younger?

What you need to know

By Robert Ebeling, D.C.

Copyright 2025

Table of Contents

4

Do you feel like you're 80 years old?

I hope not. But if you do, I want you to know—there *are* things you can do to change that.

Feeling young, energized, and full of life is what health is really about. It's what we all want, especially when we feel like we've lost it. Living a life where you can pursue your goals without being held back by "aches and pains" often chalked up to "just getting older" is not only possible—it's worth striving for.

Yes, we all age. But how we *feel* as we age varies dramatically. Some people push through pain because they're tough, or because they have no choice—they're responsible for others and just keep going. But how much better would life be if you didn't have to push through pain at all?

When it comes to whether you feel 80 or 25, there are three areas we need to look at: physical, chemical, and emotional health.

Some of these are within your control—your daily habits, your choices. 1What aren't you doing that your body needs? What are you doing that could be holding you back?

And yes, some things might seem beyond your control, like your genetics or family history—but you might be surprised by how much can be improved when you know what to look for.

In this book, I'll walk you through the key areas of your health, explain why they matter, and show you what you can do to stop feeling like you're 80—and start living the life you want.

Why do you feel like you're 80?

Likely, it's because your body hurts—not just a little, but a lot, and on a daily basis. You wake up in the morning and instead of jumping out of bed ready to go, you groan and think, *"Do I really have to do this?"* or *"What's going to hurt today?"*

Maybe you have nagging injuries contributing to your pain: shoulders and knees from playing sports; a whiplash injury from one or more car crashes; lower back trouble from heavy lifting; or repetitive motions from work. These are the obvious traumas most people recognize.

But there are other injuries we don't usually associate with chronic pain. Surgery, for example, is a major trauma to the body with long-lasting effects. Even though you were under anesthesia and you "recovered," your body still remembers it. The same is true for other procedures—root canals, mammograms, C-sections, breast implants, hair transplants, and more. If you were "cut on," that was a trauma, and it leaves a lasting imprint.

Even childhood injuries like broken bones matter. Sure, the cast came off after six to eight weeks and you were told you were "healed," but the nervous system still carries that memory. Or maybe it's something you've completely forgotten about—like a fall off a ladder five years ago.

You might be thinking, *"That was 20 years ago—it doesn't matter."* But it does. The memory of that injury is still there, quietly lurking in your nervous system.

There are also the slow, silent injuries—from working at a computer eight hours a day, or constantly looking down at your phone. Gravity never takes a day off, and your posture pays the price. You've probably seen teenagers hunched over their iPhones scrolling through social media.

You might not feel the effects now, but over time, it adds up. Your mom was right—posture matters.

But really, it's not just the pain that makes us feel 80. It's the things we can no longer do—the activities we've had to give up, the experiences we're missing out on. That's what makes us feel old and we want our lives back.

Other not so obvious reasons we can feel like we're 80

It's not just physical injuries that can make us feel old—our lifestyle plays a huge role, too. The food we eat, our (nonexistent?) exercise habits, whether we smoke or vape, how well we sleep, the emotional stress we carry from work or family, alcohol use (or abuse), coffee intake, vitamin deficiencies, digestion issues, toxin buildup, chronic inflammation (a big one!), side effects from medications, and even our DNA—all of these can contribute to feeling much older than we are.

DNA, in particular, is such a powerful factor in how our bodies function—and how we feel—that it's the first thing I want to dig into.

How our lives begin with DNA

So let's start at the beginning. How did we get here? Well, it's all about Chemistry! You came to be through a unique exchange of genetic material from your mother and father.

Don't worry if this next part sounds a little technical—it's just a simple overview so the rest of the book makes more sense.

I want you to understand the "Big Picture" of DNA and why it's important.

You've probably seen a picture of DNA. The double helix model from books that looks rather complicated because it can be. The 23 pairs of chromosomes that you have are a complex chemical structure; that if it was unraveled, would actually resemble a ladder.

The two sides of the ladder are each made up of a long chain of a sugar and a phosphate molecule. These combine together all the way down and it keeps repeating the same sequence. Each rung of the ladder has a pair of 4 possible chemical structures called nucleotides. Each nucleotide is a molecule made up of a nitrogen base, and depending on the structure, it becomes one of four types: A, T, C, or G.

In DNA these are Guanine (G), Cytosine (C), Adenine (A), and Thymine (T). Normally (G) and (C) from above will pair up as will (A) and (T) on the ladder rungs.

So you see, your DNA is just chemistry! And that's all you need to know about it for now.

Now your DNA Chromosomes have sections in them that make up genes. The purpose of a gene is to make the enzymes and other chemicals that run your body's chemistry.

When we talk about a gene, we're usually looking at just one side of the DNA strand (or one side of the ladder)— the 'coding' strand—since that's where the instructions are written. If we looked at it closely it might look something like this: GAAAGCGCTC (the first letter of the nucleotides).

Anyway, sometimes in the gene you'll get something "different" and you will "be different" from other people, and of course that's what's gives us such a diverse population with different characteristics.

Some of the "differences" are good; however some are not beneficial at all. For example, maybe you got the gene that predisposes you to getting Rheumatoid arthritis and because of lifestyle or other environmental factors it is now manifesting in your life experience.

Or maybe you don't convert folic acid very well from its "dietary" form to its "methylated" form. (The one that's actually needed inside the body to run the body processes). A lot of people understand this when they say they have the "MTHFR gene".

These examples might make you feel like you're 80 years old. But again, there are things you can do. We'll talk more about this later.

Where does our Energy come from?

Not having the energy we once did can make us feel like we're 80 years old. Chronic fatigue is a common symptom for people dealing with infections, immune system imbalances, and even certain genetic variations.[1,2,3] *(Another good reason to consider DNA testing.)*

Inside every cell, you have tiny energy factories called mitochondria. They're responsible for producing your body's energy through a process called the **Krebs cycle**—a series of chemical reactions that convert nutrients into usable energy. Since this cycle involves many steps, there are multiple opportunities for things to go wrong. If any part of it is disrupted, the result can be low energy.

After the Krebs cycle, the process continues into what's called the **Electron Transport Chain**, also inside the mitochondria. This is where your body produces **ATP**—the actual fuel your cells use to function. Unfortunately, inflammation and toxins—especially from heavy metals—can severely disrupt this energy-making process.

I still remember learning about the Krebs cycle in college chemistry. What surprised me most was discovering that **fluoride**—a common environmental toxin—can interfere with energy production. Yet fluoride is added to our drinking water and found in most toothpastes, which we're told to use multiple times a day.

And if you've ever looked at a toothpaste label, you might have noticed a warning: *"If more than used for brushing is accidentally swallowed, get medical help or contact a Poison Control Center right away."* That's because fluoride, in high enough doses, is toxic.

Now imagine if we could tap into the same energy we had as kids—how much more we could get done! I can't help but wonder if over time, we've built up an accumulation of fluoride and other toxins that's contributing to our declining energy.

No wonder so many people turn to coffee just to get through the day. But while caffeine gives us a temporary boost, it's not creating new energy—it's just shifting how we use it. I think of Einstein's quote: *"Energy cannot be created or destroyed, only transformed."*

Coffee stimulates the adrenal glands, giving us a temporary push, but eventually, we have to pay for that burst—with more fatigue, more aches, and potentially more health problems.

And one more note—most conventionally grown coffee is heavily treated with pesticides (up to 250 pounds per acre!). So if you do enjoy coffee, I recommend choosing organic whenever possible.

Why do we get sick?

Your immune system is designed to protect you from foreign invaders like bacteria and viruses. When it's strong, it fights off infections quickly. But when it's **weakened**—due to poor nutrition, lack of sleep, chronic stress, or habits like smoking—you're more likely to get sick (4). Even your **DNA** can influence how well your immune system works.

When you do get sick, your body launches an inflammatory response. This is why you might experience **fever, pain,** or **swelling**—it's actually your body trying to heal. So inflammation, in the short term, is a **normal and necessary** part of getting well.

The problem starts when inflammation sticks around. **Chronic inflammation**—that is, inflammation that doesn't go away—can be a sign of an **autoimmune condition**, where the body mistakenly attacks its own tissues (5).

Several chemicals drive the inflammatory process. The most well-known are:

- **Prostaglandins** – involved in pain and fever.
- **Histamine** – released by mast cells and basophils, especially during allergic reactions.
- **Cytokines** – chemical messengers that coordinate immune responses.
- **Bradykinins** – cause blood vessels to widen and create pain.
- **Leukotrienes** – inflammatory compounds made from a fatty acid called arachidonic acid (6).

Speaking of fatty acids—your **diet** has a major impact on inflammation. The balance between **Omega-3** and **Omega-6** fatty acids is especially important.

- **Omega-3s** (found in fish oil, flaxseed oil, and walnut oil) are **anti-inflammatory**.
- **Too many Omega-6s** (found in many processed vegetable oils) can be **pro-inflammatory**.

Histamine, a key player in inflammation, is broken down by your body using nutrients like **vitamin B6, methylated folate (the active form of folic acid)**, and **vitamin C**. If your body can't clear histamine properly, it may build up and worsen inflammation.

And if you've got too much inflammation going on—you guessed it—it can make you feel like you're 80 years old all over again!

Free radicals and the Aging Process

What Is a Free Radical?

Free radicals are **highly reactive molecules** that can damage your body's cells and tissues. One of the most common types is based on **oxygen**, and these are often referred to as **reactive oxygen species (ROS)**.

Free radicals are unstable because they have **an unpaired electron**, which makes them eager to react with other molecules—like your **DNA**, **RNA**, or **proteins**—causing damage in the process.

Another example is a nitrogen-based free radical called **nitric oxide**, which also plays a role in inflammation and oxidative stress.

Where Do Free Radicals Come From?

Your body produces free radicals from both **internal processes** and **external exposures**.

Internal Sources:

- **Normal metabolism**
  Your body naturally produces free radicals during energy production—especially inside your mitochondria.
- **Enzyme activity**
  Certain immune cells, like white blood cells, use enzyme reactions to kill invading bacteria. One way they do this is by releasing **hypochlorite** (yes, the same chemical used in bleach!) to rupture the membranes of harmful microbes.

- **Inflammation and immune responses**
  When your immune system is active or inflamed, it can increase free radical production.
- **Intense exercise**
  Heavy physical exertion increases oxygen demand and metabolic activity, which can also spike free radical output.

External Sources:

- **Environmental pollution**
  Breathing in air pollutants, ozone, or chemical toxins can boost free radical levels.
- **Radiation exposure**
  X-rays, ultraviolet (UV) rays from the sun, and other forms of radiation can lead to free radical formation.
- **Cigarette smoke**
  Tobacco smoke contains hundreds of harmful chemicals that contribute to oxidative stress. In fact cigarette smoking has now been linked as a cause of developing Rheumatoid arthritis, the most common inflammatory arthritic condition.
- **Certain drugs and industrial chemicals**
  Exposure to pesticides, solvents, or medications can increase free radical production.
- **Dietary factors**
  Highly processed foods, excess sugar, and unhealthy fats can all influence oxidative stress in the body (7).

When too many free radicals build up—and your body doesn't have the tools to get rid of them—it leads to **oxidative stress**. That kind of cellular damage not only accelerates aging... it can absolutely make you feel like you're 80 years old.

What are you eating and are you digesting?

I've read the book *4 Blood Types, 4 Diets, Eat Right 4 Your Type* by Dr. Peter D'Adamo a few times. It explores how your blood type can influence how you respond to certain foods, and how eating according to your type could help improve health and prevent disease. Although the medical community has pushed back against it, I think it makes a lot of sense.

Here's a brief summary:

- **Type O** – the oldest and most common blood type. A high-protein diet is recommended, with an emphasis on avoiding grains, beans, legumes, and dairy.
- **Type A** – the second most common. A vegetarian diet is best suited here.
- **Type B** – generally can eat a wide variety of foods without restriction.
- **Type AB** – more of a "Mediterranean-style" approach, including dairy, lamb, fish, grains, fruits, and vegetables.

A key takeaway for Type O individuals is to avoid both dairy and gluten, as they're common allergens. Gluten is also notorious for contributing to weight gain—so no beer or wheat pasta for Type O.

Speaking of weight gain, if you're trying to lose weight, your diet plays a more critical role than exercise. Excess weight puts strain on your knees, hips, and lower back. Being overweight can make you feel decades older and increases your risk for future joint replacements.

If you're interested in the details, I'd recommend picking up a copy of the book.

Another important topic is **histamine**, which is the third most common source of inflammation in the body (after old injuries and fatty acid imbalances). Inflammation can lead to weakness in key muscles due to muscle-organ relationships. For example, the quadriceps are associated with the small intestines—the site where nutrient absorption happens.

Are you unknowingly consuming histamine-rich foods? Some common culprits include:

- Aged cheese
- Eggplant
- Tomatoes
- Chocolate
- Processed meats
- Beer and wine
- Eggs
- Fermented foods
- Shellfish
- Spinach
- Strawberries
- Dairy
- Peanuts
- Avocados
- Pickled or canned foods

(Whew! After reading that list, you might be wondering what's left to eat.)

How well is your digestive system functioning? As we age, our bodies produce fewer digestive enzymes—from the pancreas, liver, gallbladder, stomach, and small intestines. Without these enzymes, food isn't properly broken down, leading to slower digestion and reduced nutrient absorption. Overeating can also overwhelm your system.

If you're consuming too much sugar regularly, you can develop **insulin resistance**, a condition where sugar no longer enters your cells effectively.

Another issue that can disrupt digestion is **yeast overgrowth**, often triggered by antibiotics that wipe out both good and bad bacteria. Yeast produces toxic aldehydes, which burden the liver. It can also damage the intestinal lining, leading to **leaky gut**—where larger, undigested particles pass through the gut wall into the bloodstream, creating more inflammation.

There's even a reflex point at the belly button that can be muscle tested to check for the presence of yeast. If it tests weak, we can evaluate various nutritional products to see what may help.

Parasites are another unwelcome guest—often contracted through contaminated food, especially raw fish like sushi. Symptoms of a parasitic infection include abdominal pain, diarrhea, vomiting, weight loss, fatigue, rashes, and itching (8). Black walnut is a common natural remedy used to address parasites.

If you're dealing with parasites or leaky gut, it's no wonder you might feel like you're 80 years old!

Why you Need Vitamins!

The word "vitamin" comes from "vital"—and that's exactly what they are: vital for your body to function properly. Minerals like **magnesium** and **zinc** are involved in over 700 different chemical reactions in the body. Everything from energy production to detoxification depends on them.

Think you're getting all the nutrients you need from your diet? Think again—especially if you follow the typical American "fast food" diet. Even if you're taking supplements (and you *should be!*), here's a question for you:

If vitamin supplements didn't exist, where would your nutrition come from?
That's right—**your food.**
So why aren't you chewing your vitamins?

(I know, they taste bad. But let's be honest—most things that are good for you usually don't taste great.)

Digestion starts in the mouth. When you chew your food—or your chewable vitamins—you begin the breakdown process. Chewing activates **saliva**, which contains digestive enzymes. The **alkaline pH** of saliva helps trigger **stomach acid production**, essential for further digestion.

Plus, your **tongue is a sensory powerhouse**—tasting nutrients sends a signal straight to your nervous system, preparing your body to absorb and use those nutrients immediately. It's a fast, efficient system—when used properly.

A high-quality multivitamin from a reputable company can act like a cheap **nutritional insurance policy**, helping cover any dietary gaps. Look for one with antioxidants like **Vitamin A, C, E, glutathione, selenium**, and the essential minerals **zinc and magnesium**.

That said, not all vitamins are created equal. Some supplements contain nutrient forms that your body can't use effectively. For example, **folic acid** and **vitamin B6** must go through a conversion process before they're usable. This process requires enzymes—and you guessed it—**other vitamins and minerals** to make it happen.

But if you're not taking *any* vitamins at all?
Then don't be surprised if you feel like you're 80 years old.

Are you Detoxing?

With all the pollution in our environment today—heavy metals in seafood, pesticides on conventionally grown crops, and toxins even in the water we drink—it's more important than ever to support your body's natural detox processes.

One simple and powerful way to do that is through **fasting**.

Fasting gives your body a much-needed break from constantly processing incoming food and toxins. When you're not digesting, your system has time to clean up what's already lingering. Even **intermittent fasting**—such as eating during an 8-hour window—can give your body time to reset. It also happens to be great for **weight loss**.

A basic intermittent fasting schedule could look like this:

- Skip breakfast (maybe just have a cup of black coffee)
- Eat your first meal around **10 a.m.**
- Lunch around **2 p.m.**
- Dinner by **6 p.m.**

You might go to bed feeling a little hungry at first—but here's the good news: you usually wake up *not* feeling hungry. That's because your body is now burning **stored fat** for energy. It might take a few days to adjust, but once you get into the rhythm, it becomes much easier.

Now, let's talk about your **liver**—the body's detox powerhouse. One of its main jobs is to **detoxify blood**, especially blood coming from your large intestines, where a lot of waste products and toxins accumulate.

For the science-minded: liver detox happens in **two phases**.

- **Phase 1** uses enzymes like *Cytochrome P450* to convert toxins into intermediate compounds.
- **Phase 2** then transforms those into water-soluble products that can be safely eliminated from the body.

Keeping your liver healthy is essential—not just for detox, but for your overall health and vitality. Because when your liver isn't functioning well, guess what? You're more likely to feel like you're 80 years old.

Why you need Water!

Your body is made up of about 60% water, and nearly every system depends on it to function properly. Water helps regulate your temperature, transport nutrients, cushion your joints, protect your organs, and—yes—flush out waste through the kidneys, liver, skin, and intestines. Without enough water, your body has to work harder, and that stress shows up in surprising ways.

One place dehydration hits hard is your **spinal discs**. These discs—the shock absorbers between your vertebrae—are made of at least 75% water (9). When you're dehydrated, your body prioritizes vital organs and may start pulling water from less critical structures like the discs. That's why people often feel **stiff, tight, or achy** when they haven't had enough to drink. Chronic dehydration can even contribute to disc degeneration over time.

Start your day with water. After 7–8 hours of sleep without fluids, your body is naturally dehydrated. A tall glass of clean water first thing in the morning helps jumpstart your metabolism, support brain function, and rehydrate your tissues. Want to feel like you're 80 years old? Skip the water and start the day with caffeine alone.

Water Quality: What Are You Really Drinking?

Not all water is created equal. While I'm not suggesting you drink distilled water (since it lacks essential minerals), it is smart to **filter your tap water**. Why? Because our municipal water systems weren't designed to deal with modern pharmaceutical waste. Many medications—birth control, antidepressants, painkillers—end up in the water supply after being excreted or flushed. Wastewater treatment plants remove many contaminants, but they're not perfect.

To illustrate the point: after water leaves your home, it's processed and released into rivers or reservoirs... and those often become the source for another city downstream. Do you really think all traces of drugs, hormones, or pesticides are gone by the time it reaches your tap again?

Just ask the residents of **Flint, Michigan**, who learned the hard way that you can't always trust government oversight to protect your water. Contaminants like lead, which is toxic even in small amounts, can have lasting health effects—especially on the nervous system.

So what should you drink? Personally, I prefer to fill my own containers at **Natural Grocers**, where they offer reverse osmosis-filtered water. It's cleaner and more affordable than most bottled options—and you're not adding more plastic to the landfill.

How Much Water Should You Drink?

Everyone's needs vary based on activity level, climate, and health, but a **good general rule** is at least **half a gallon (64 oz) per day**. If you're very active, sweat a lot, or live at high altitude, you may need more. And remember, by the time you feel thirsty, you're already mildly dehydrated.

If you are not drinking water because it "has no taste", try adding a pinch of sea salt to it. It has electrolytes your body needs and makes it more palatable as well.

Pro tip: If you're getting headaches, constipation, fatigue, or dry skin—it may not be a lack of vitamins, it might just be a lack of water.

Do you exercise?

Remember back in grade school when you had mandatory P.E. class? Ever wonder why that was required? They were trying to teach you the importance of **daily physical activity**—and just because you graduated doesn't mean you're off the hook now!

Are you moving your body beyond what's required at work? If not, you're asking for trouble. Exercise—especially **cardiovascular activity**—boosts endurance, energy, circulation, and detoxification. It sends oxygen-rich blood to every part of the body and helps regenerate and repair tissue.

It also prevents **muscle atrophy**. Look at elderly people who've lost a lot of muscle mass. That doesn't just happen because of age—it happens because of **inactivity**. If you don't want to feel or look like you're 80 years old, you need to be **exercising regularly**.

Cardio workouts, like **walking** or **biking**, are excellent for boosting your metabolism and burning body fat—as long as you stay in the **aerobic zone**. What does that mean? You should still be able to carry on a conversation while exercising. If you're gasping for breath, you've shifted into **anaerobic mode**, which burns sugar instead of fat.

Don't forget about **stretching**! It's a great way to feel younger and stay flexible. Sitting at a desk all week? That's not doing your muscles any favors. In fact, **sitting is now considered the "new smoking"**—it leads to tight, rigid muscles from staying in the same position for too long.

One of the best stretches I've ever done is called the **groin stretch**. It doesn't look like much at first, but it's powerful—and yes, it *hurts* in a good way. Here's how to do it:

- Lie flat on your back with one leg resting on a box or sturdy chair.
- The elevated leg should be bent at **90 degrees** at the hip, knee, and ankle.
- The other leg stays straight on the floor with the ankle flexed at 90 degrees, pointing straight up.
- Hold this position for **20 minutes**—then switch sides and do the other leg for 20 more.

Yes, it's a long stretch, but try it once and feel the difference. You'll thank me later.

Another fantastic stretch for your **hamstrings** is done sitting on the floor with your back against a wall and your legs straight in front of you. Want a trick to make it more effective? **Contract your quadriceps**—forcefully squeezing your quads sends a signal to your brain to relax the opposing muscles (your hamstrings). This **neurological trick** helps the hamstrings let go, so you get a deeper, safer stretch.

So carve out some time each week—at least on the weekends—to do some stretching.

Because **not stretching**? That's one of the fastest ways to start feeling like you're 80 years old.

Why you Need Sleep!

Sleep: Your Overnight Repair Shop

We spend about **one-third of our lives sleeping**—and for good reason. Sleep isn't just "time off." It's when your body shifts into deep **recovery and repair mode**, restoring everything from your muscles to your immune system.

You need about **8 hours of quality sleep** each night. Not just to feel rested, but because this is when your **brain does its housecleaning**. While you sleep, your brain activates a process called the **glymphatic system**, which flushes out metabolic waste—including a substance called **beta-amyloid**. When beta-amyloid builds up, it forms plaques in the brain, and this accumulation has been strongly associated with **Alzheimer's disease**.

Let that sink in: sleep isn't just about energy. It could play a **major role in preventing neurodegeneration**.

And here's something empowering—**your DNA test can tell you** if you carry genes associated with a higher risk for Alzheimer's (like the **APOE-e4 variant**). That doesn't mean you're doomed—it means you have the chance to **intervene early** with lifestyle changes, like improving sleep, reducing inflammation, and optimizing brain health.

Better to know now and take action than to find out when it's too late.

If you don't sleep well, not only will you **feel like you're 80**—you'll **age like it too**.

Doctor's tip: **Sleep on your back or your side, but not on your stomach. Stomach sleeping is one sure way to wake up with your back and neck hurting and make you feel like you're 80 years old!**

Setting Up Your Sleep Environment

To get the most out of sleep, your **environment matters.** Your bedroom should be **completely dark**—and I mean pitch black. Even small lights from a **GFCI outlet, alarm clock, modem, router**, or your phone charger can disrupt your brain's production of **melatonin**, your body's natural sleep hormone.

Solutions:

- Cover light sources with **black electrical tape**
- Unplug or relocate devices that emit light
- Use **blackout curtains** if outside light seeps in
- If full darkness isn't possible, wear a comfortable **sleep mask**

Also, avoid **blue light** for at least an hour before bed. That means no phones, tablets, TVs, or laptops. Blue light signals your brain that it's daytime, **shutting down melatonin production** and making it harder to fall (and stay) asleep.

Why Melatonin Matters

Melatonin isn't just about sleep—it's also a **potent antioxidant**. That means it helps neutralize **free radicals**, those unstable molecules that damage cells and accelerate aging.

So if you're cutting your sleep short or staying up late staring at screens, you're not just losing rest—you're losing one of your body's best natural defenses.

Bottom Line

Prioritize sleep like your life depends on it—because it kind of does. Aging faster, thinking slower, gaining weight, feeling anxious, and even developing chronic diseases are all linked to **poor sleep habits**.

Want to feel 40 when you're 80? Get your 8 hours of sleep.

The Immune System

Strengthening Your Immune System: Nutrients and Glands

One of the **most important nutrients** for your immune system is **Vitamin D**. This vitamin is unique in that it can be produced by your body in response to **sunlight exposure**. Unlike melatonin, which thrives in darkness to promote sleep, Vitamin D is synthesized when your skin is exposed to the sun. That's why it's so important to get **outside** for at least **20 minutes each morning** to help set your body's internal clock. This boosts not only your immune system but also supports a healthy **sleep-wake cycle**.

The Key Immune System Glands: Thymus and Spleen

Your immune system depends on the proper functioning of several key organs and glands, two of the most important being the **Thymus** and **Spleen**.

1. **The Thymus Gland:**
   Located beneath your sternum, close to your heart, the thymus is critical for the production of **T-cells**, which help fight off **viruses** and **cancer cells**. A fascinating way to support your thymus is by massaging the reflex area near your right rib cage, just below the armpit. When your thymus needs support, this area can become **tender**. The thymus also responds well to **Zinc**, a vital nutrient for immune function.
2. **The Spleen:**
   Located on the left side of your body, the spleen acts like a **filtration system** for your blood. It removes **dead and dying red blood cells**, recycling them into **iron** and **bilirubin**. These red blood cells are responsible for transporting **oxygen** and **nutrients** throughout your body, and they typically live for about 120 days. To support the spleen, **Vitamin C** is an excellent nutrient to keep in your diet—it not only aids the spleen but also helps **detoxify histamines**.

Immune System Reflex Areas

There are **three primary reflex points** in the body related to immune system function:

1. **Thymus Reflex (Right Rib Cage):**
   As mentioned, the area around the right rib cage is linked to the thymus. Tenderness here can indicate a need for support, and Zinc is particularly helpful.
2. **Spleen Reflex (Left Rib Cage):**
   The left side of the body houses the spleen, and there's also a reflex point there. If it feels sensitive, it might indicate the spleen needs attention. **Vitamin C** and other antioxidants are key nutrients for this area.

3. **Chemical Sensitivities (Lower Sternum):**
   This reflex area is tied to **detoxification** issues in the body. If you're sensitive to substances like cigarette smoke, perfumes, or chemicals, your body might be struggling with **detoxification**. In such cases, the trace mineral **molybdenum** can help your system clear out these toxins. People with heavy metal toxicity often experience symptoms in this region as well, which can affect the **Krebs cycle**—the energy production process in your cells.

The Role of Heavy Metals in Immune Health

Heavy metals, such as **lead**, **mercury**, and **cadmium**, can disrupt your immune system and energy production. These metals tend to accumulate in the **salivary glands**, which filter fluids to create saliva. You can even test for the presence of heavy metals using **muscle testing**. Have the person swish a small amount of saliva in their mouth, and see if it weakens their muscle strength. If so, **molybdenum** or **alpha-lipoic acid** (which supports the Krebs cycle and contains sulfur) may help strengthen the body.

Zinc is another powerful mineral to help detoxify heavy metals, and there are also **reflex points behind the collarbone** that can indicate the presence of toxins. If pressing these points weakens a muscle, it could be a sign of heavy metal toxicity. Additionally, **the Pectoralis Minor muscle** tends to weaken in the presence of these metals, which can also signal an issue.

Autoimmunity: When the Immune System Attacks Itself

Sometimes, the immune system doesn't just fight off invaders—it **turns on the body** itself. This is known as

autoimmune disease, and it occurs when the immune system mistakenly attacks its own tissues. Conditions like **Rheumatoid arthritis**, **Hypothyroidism**, and many others are linked to an overactive immune response.

Managing autoimmune diseases often requires **immune system modifications**, proper nutrition, and addressing underlying stressors like inflammation or toxin buildup. By focusing on things like **Vitamin D**, **Zinc**, and **antioxidants**, you can help regulate immune function and support overall health.

Bottom Line: Supporting Your Immune System Naturally

The immune system is a complex network that relies on **proper nutrition, glandular health**, and **detoxification** to function at its best. By understanding the role of the **Thymus**, **Spleen**, and **reflex areas**, and by supporting them with the right nutrients like **Vitamin D**, **Zinc**, and **Vitamin C**, you can **optimize immune function** and protect yourself from a range of diseases.

Don't forget: **heavy metals** and **chemical sensitivities** also play a role in immune health. By being proactive about detoxification and using **natural remedies** like **molybdenum** and **alpha-lipoic acid**, you can help your body fight off toxins before they get the best of you.

The Endocrine system

The Endocrine System: Hormones and Muscle Relationships

The **endocrine system** plays a crucial role in regulating hormones that affect nearly every function in the body. Key components of the endocrine system include the **pituitary gland, pineal gland, thyroid, parathyroid, adrenal glands**, and **reproductive organs** (ovaries/uterus in women; prostate/testicles in men). Each of these glands produces hormones that influence everything from growth and metabolism to mood and energy levels.

As you probably know, **hormones** can dramatically affect how you feel and act. A small imbalance in hormone production can have a big impact on your health and overall well-being.

Muscle/Organ Relationships in the Endocrine System

One of the most fascinating aspects of the body is how the **muscles** are directly linked to specific **organs and glands** in the endocrine system. These muscle/organ relationships are a key to understanding certain muscle weaknesses and underlying endocrine issues. Here are a few critical connections:

- **Teres Minor/Thyroid**
- **Sartorius and Gracilis/Adrenals**
- **Gluteus Medius/Reproductive System**

For example, if you experience **weakness in the Teres Minor muscle** (part of the rotator cuff in the shoulder); it might indicate a **shoulder pain** issue. However, this weakness could also be a sign of an **underactive thyroid**. The thyroid gland, which regulates metabolism and energy production, can affect muscle strength and function. So, in cases of muscle weakness, it's important to consider the possibility that an **endocrine problem** might be contributing to the issue.

Adrenal Fatigue: The Common Culprit

Among the most common endocrine issues people experience are problems with the **adrenal glands**, which produce adrenaline and cortisol in response to stress.

Stress is a natural response that can be beneficial in small doses, helping you face challenges. However, **chronic stress**—whether from **mental**, **physical**, or **chemical** sources—can overwhelm your adrenal glands, leading to **adrenal fatigue**.

Some common sources of stress include:

- **Mental stress**: Relationship issues, work pressure, financial worries.
- **Physical stress**: Injuries, overexertion, lack of sleep.
- **Chemical stress**: Poor diet (too much sugar or caffeine) or exposure to toxins.

When your adrenal glands are overworked, they can impact your body's **energy** levels and **muscle function**. One of the reasons people with **lower back** or **knee pain** often have adrenal issues is because the muscles associated with the adrenal glands (particularly those that run from the pelvis down to the knee) aren't functioning correctly. These muscles become weak, which can make it harder for your body to properly support the lower back or knees.

If you're dealing with **adrenal fatigue**, you may also experience symptoms like **feeling lightheaded** when standing up too quickly. This happens because the adrenal glands help regulate **blood pressure** when you change positions. If your adrenals aren't functioning properly, it becomes harder for your body to adjust to these changes, resulting in dizziness or lightheadedness.

Hormone Imbalances: Feeling Older Than Your Age

When your **hormones** aren't balanced, it can make you feel like you're aging faster than you should. You may not feel like you're 80, but you might notice symptoms that make you feel much older than your actual age—fatigue, muscle weakness, joint pain, and difficulty managing stress.

Getting your **endocrine system** back on track is essential to feeling your best and maintaining energy and vitality. Whether through nutrition, stress management, or targeted treatments, supporting your adrenal glands, thyroid, and other key hormones can make a significant difference in how you feel every day.

Muscle Testing for Endocrine Imbalances

One valuable tool for understanding endocrine imbalances is **muscle testing**. By muscle testing, we can identify why a specific muscle is weak and determine what it may respond to—whether it's a nutritional supplement, a glandular issue, or other underlying health concern.

The Emotional System

The Emotional Connection to Health

In Chinese medicine, emotions are considered a primary cause of many health problems. Different emotions are believed to target specific organs, and understanding this connection can offer insight into how emotional health impacts your physical well-being.

For instance:

- **Anger** is commonly associated with the **liver** in men.
- **Worry** is often linked to the **stomach** in women.

Consider the role of the **liver**—it produces **bile**, which is essential for digesting fats, and stores it in the **gall bladder** for when it's needed. Now, think about how **anger** or unresolved anger gets stored in the body. What does that emotion become if left unaddressed? **Resentment**. Over time, **resentment** can disrupt liver function, leading to issues with the gall bladder.

Similarly, **grief** is often connected to the **lungs**. That's why it's not uncommon for someone who has lost a long-term partner to develop severe lung conditions, such as **pneumonia**, shortly after the loss. Grief literally affects the respiratory system, and emotions tied to loss can manifest physically in the body.

The Toll of Toxic Relationships

Speaking of emotional stress, one of the most debilitating experiences is being stuck in a **toxic relationship**, especially with a **narcissist**. These relationships can drain your mental and physical health, and sometimes the best choice for your well-being is to **leave**.

There's a piece of advice I once heard that resonates with many aspects of life: **"If you want an easy life, do the hard thing. If you want a hard life, do the easy thing."** This is particularly true when it comes to unhealthy relationships. Staying in a toxic situation might seem easier in the short term, but the emotional and physical toll can make life far more difficult in the long run.

Treating Emotional Conditions Quickly

For those dealing with emotional struggles like **stress, worry, anxiety,** or **depression**, Chinese medicine offers a technique for **quick emotional relief**. There are specific reflex points located across the front of the forehead that can be muscle-tested and treated by tapping on them. This practice can help release emotional blockages and promote a sense of well-being. Many people find it helpful for addressing immediate emotional challenges.

Emotional health is just as important as physical health, and an abundance of unresolved emotional issues can contribute to **premature aging**. Chronic stress and emotional turmoil can wear you down faster than you might realize—making you feel older than your actual age.

Cartilage regeneration

Cartilage Regeneration: How Your Body Repairs Itself

Your body has the remarkable ability to repair its own cartilage. However, there are key factors that can influence this process, and some things can actually hinder the body's natural cartilage regeneration.

1. The Impact of Medications and Diet
Chronic use of **Non-Steroidal Anti-Inflammatory Drugs (NSAIDs)**—like **aspirin, acetaminophen**, and similar painkillers—can block the body's ability to regenerate cartilage. While these medications can provide temporary relief from pain, they can interfere with the body's natural healing processes, especially when used over long periods of time.

Another major factor that impedes cartilage repair is **sugar**. High sugar intake can contribute to inflammation, which disrupts the body's ability to repair damaged tissue, including cartilage. Therefore, limiting sugar in your diet can support better cartilage health and overall joint function.

2. Sulfur: A Key Nutrient for Cartilage Regeneration
Sulfur is an essential nutrient in the synthesis of cartilage. It is involved in the production of collagen, a key structural protein in cartilage. If your body is low in sulfur or if heavy metals are binding to the sulfur in your system, it can significantly hinder the process of cartilage regeneration. Heavy metal toxicity—such as from lead or mercury—can interfere with many bodily functions, including the regeneration of cartilage.

3. The Effect of Obesity and Joint Strain
Carrying excess weight puts a tremendous amount of strain on your joints, especially the **knees**, **hips**, and **lower back**. The added pressure accelerates the wear and tear of cartilage, leading to premature degeneration and pain. Obesity is a major contributor to joint problems because it increases the stress on cartilage, often causing irreversible damage over time.

4. When Cartilage Repair Isn't Enough
In some cases, cartilage degeneration is so severe that the body's natural repair mechanisms can't keep up. When this happens, more **aggressive interventions** may be necessary. **Stem cell therapy** can provide a potential solution, offering the possibility of regenerating damaged cartilage. However, for many people, **surgery** or even **joint replacement** may become the only option.

The Consequences of Cartilage Damage

Experiencing the effects of damaged cartilage can make you feel much older than your actual age. Nothing can make you feel like you're **80 years old** more than having the physical limitations and joint pain that often accompany severe cartilage degeneration.

Other Factors you were unaware of

Understanding DNA and Its Impact on Health

One often overlooked factor in your health is your **DNA mutations**, also known as **SNPs** (Single Nucleotide Polymorphisms). Simply put, **SNPs** refer to a change in the nucleotide at a specific location in the DNA. This change can affect how your body functions, and it's crucial to understand how these mutations can influence your health.

As we discussed earlier, your **body chemistry** is essentially a series of biochemical reactions that convert one substance into another. These reactions are regulated by **enzymes**, which are proteins your body produces. And guess what? The **instructions** for creating these enzymes come from your **DNA**.

Your **DNA** contains **genes**, and each gene has specific instructions for making the enzymes necessary for these processes. Think of it as the written **blueprint** for how your body operates. For instance, enzymes are needed to create neurotransmitters, which are responsible for brain function. The enzymes involved in these processes are determined by the genetic code your body carries—essentially, you are the product of your parents' DNA, and it shapes your unique body chemistry.

How DNA Mutations Affect Your Health

If you have **mutations** in your DNA, these can help explain why you might struggle with certain health conditions. For example, not producing enough of a particular enzyme or producing too much can lead to issues with metabolism, mood, and energy levels. These enzyme imbalances can also affect how you interact with the world and the people around you.

Some common health concerns that may be linked to your DNA include:

- **Allergies and Gluten Sensitivities**: DNA analysis can reveal if you have genetic markers that predispose you to sensitivities or allergies.
- **Mental Health Conditions**: Conditions like **depression, anxiety, bipolar disorder**, and **brain fog** can all be influenced by genetic factors. Key genes like **MAO** (monoamine oxidase) and **COMT** (catechol-O-methyltransferase) play critical roles in regulating neurotransmitters such as **serotonin, dopamine, epinephrine**, and **norepinephrine**. If these genes are mutated, it can disrupt the balance of brain chemicals, leading to mood swings and stress perception issues.
- **Energy Problems**: DNA mutations can also affect how efficiently your body produces **ATP**, the energy currency of your cells. If your ATP production is inefficient, it can lead to chronic fatigue and other energy-related problems.
- **Sleep Disorders**: Many people struggle with sleep, and your DNA can offer insight into why. The process of converting **serotonin** into **melatonin**, which regulates your sleep cycle, is controlled by specific genes. Mutations in these genes can impact how well you sleep, leading to insomnia or poor-quality rest.

- **Sickness and Inflammation**: DNA analysis can also reveal genetic markers related to inflammation, which is often the root cause of chronic conditions like arthritis, cardiovascular disease, and autoimmune disorders.

A Quick Way to Remember

If you're feeling overwhelmed by chronic health issues, it might be time to consider a **DNA analysis**. To help my patients remember how DNA can affect their health, I use this mnemonic: **"A MESS"**.

- A for **Allergies** and **Gluten Sensitivities**
- M for **Mental Health** (depression, anxiety, etc.)
- E for **Energy Issues**
- S for **Sleep Disorders**
- S for **Sickness and Inflammation**

So if you feel like your health is "A MESS" and like you're 80 years old then your DNA could hold the answers. It's worth considering a test to uncover how your genetic makeup might be influencing your health.

The Nervous System

The Master Computer that Runs Your Entire Body

Your nervous system consists of the brain, the spinal cord (which exits the bottom of the skull and travels through your spinal column), all the nerves that come off the spinal cord, and then all the muscles and organs of the body that those nerves go to.

So in essence, your entire body is part of the nervous system.

The nervous system connects everything you do from thinking and feeling; to moving and digestion; from the beat of your heart to you taking in a breath of fresh air. Without the nervous system you wouldn't be alive, that's how important it is.

The Cranial Nerves: Specialized Nerves that are in your head

There are also 12 pairs of cranial nerves (meaning there is a right and left nerve) that come directly off the brain and have specialized functions. They include:

- **Optic Nerve**- lets you see
- **Olfactory Nerve**- lets you smell
- **Oculomotor Nerve**- lets you move your eyes
- **Trochlear Nerve**- also lets you move your eyes
- **Trigeminal Nerve**- provides motor and sensory to the face
- **Abducens Nerve**- lets you move your eyes
- **Facial Nerve**- Provides motor and sensory to the face
- **Acoustic nerve**- allows you to hear sounds
- **Glossopharyngeal Nerve-** provides sensory to the tongue, motor to the throat, and some autonomic to salivary glands.
- **Vagus Nerve**- provides motor and sensory to the gut and heart
- **Spinal Accessory Nerve**- provides motor function to the trapezius muscle
- **Hypoglossal Nerve**- provides motor function to the tongue

A simple way to understand this Important and Complex area of Your Body

When you think about it, your nervous system does basically only 2 things: it collects sensory information (like pain, temperature, touch, taste, sound, sight, smells, vibration, etc.) and then it decides what to do with that information in the form of a muscle contraction.

Some examples of that would be you touch a hot stove and you get that muscle response; you put some food in your mouth (you taste it and chew it) and you get saliva production (a motor response); someone tells you a funny joke (you hear it), you laugh (again, a motor response); you eat something bad (your gut senses it), and you throw up (a motor response).

- <u>**The previous paragraph is the most important concept in this whole book. If you understand this, then you will understand muscle testing.**</u>

Another example could be you're sitting in a doctor's office and he checks your knee reflex. A sensory stimulation (the reflex hammer hitting your knee) causes a muscle response (your knee to give a slight jerk motion).

So it's all about **sensory in and motor out**. Got it? The nervous system controls everything in your body.

The Cerebellum

Another important part of the nervous system is called the Cerebellum which is responsible for the unconscious control of your posture, balance and equilibrium. It sits in the back part of your skull and if you put your hand on the back of your head you'd be touching it.

The Cerebellum receives sensory input from a variety of places in the body. It's also the place that memory of previous injuries gets stored.

Yes, Injuries Affect the Nervous System. Let that sink in.

The brain stores the memory of that pain as a protective mechanism—a way to remind us not to repeat harmful actions. In clinical observation that pain memory gets stored on the same side as the injury. So if you had a broken arm on the right side, that injury gets recorded in the cerebellum, but in this case only on the right side and not the left.

Over time, injuries stored in the cerebellum can have lasting effects on your body. This is because the Cerebellum sends motor output to your body and it bases that output off of what sensory information it receives or is stored there. So if you have an imbalance of sensory information in the Cerebellum, the motor output will be unbalanced as well. This is one reason why as people age they have a higher risk of falls from losing their balance; too many lifetime injuries.

Emotional traumas may also lodge their effects in the Cerebellum affecting posture, balance, and equilibrium. It takes identifying the emotional trauma while muscle testing to be able to start removing its effects and restore balance to the nervous system.

The Autonomic Nervous System

The Autonomic or "Automatic" nervous system runs things in your body without you having to think about them. Things like your heart beat or your digestion.

There are 2 parts of the Autonomic system; one is called the Sympathetic and the other is the Parasympathetic. You don't need to remember their names—just know they work together to keep your body in balance. One is like the gas pedal on your car and makes things go. The other is like the brakes and slows things down when needed.

The sympathetic nervous system has its origins in the spinal cord from the Thoracic spine (middle back) down to the upper Lumbar spine (lower back). It's mostly involved with the fight or flight mechanism of the body.

The Parasympathetic nervous system is more about "rest and digest". It has its origins in the sacral part of the spine as well as some cranial nerves. One of the most important cranial nerves of the Parasympathetic nervous system is the Vagus Nerve which travels from the brain, down into the neck, and to all of your internal organs, including the heart.

Cranial Nerves are part of the Autonomic Nervous System

Sometimes we test the cranial nerves when we want to see what's going on with the Autonomic nervous system. For example, we can use the eyes while muscle testing.

Looking at something close by involves using the parasympathetic nervous system, while looking at something far away uses the sympathetic nervous system.

How this changes the outcome of a muscle test can tell us more about what's going on with the body with regards to imbalances in the Autonomic nervous system. These imbalances will tell us if the body needs more sympathetic or parasympathetic stimulation.

How problems in the nervous system can make you feel like you're 80 years old

Since the nervous system controls nearly every single function in your body, it makes sense that injuries—whether physical, emotional, or chemical—will ultimately determine how young or old you feel. Again, this is because your nervous system is all about sensory in and motor out. You fix the sensory, it fixes the motor. You fix the motor, it fixes how well your body runs.

That's the foundation. Now that you understand how your body works, it's time to shift gears.

In Part 2, we're going to explore what you can actually _do_ about it—simple, powerful strategies to start reclaiming control over how your body feels and functions, so you don't have to live like you're 80 before your time.

PART 2

What Are the Possible Solutions?

Now that you know what can make you feel like you're 80 years old, what can you do? Well, you have a wide range of options when it comes to dealing with pain, injuries, or chronic discomfort. Let's break them down:

Option A: Do Nothing and Ignore the Problem

This might seem like the easiest path—but it's often the worst. Most problems, especially physical injuries like those from a whiplash-type car crash, tend to get worse over time. Left unaddressed, inflammation can lead to degeneration, arthritis, and permanent damage.

Option B: Do at Home Therapy: Ice or Heat?

But which should you use—ice or heat?

- **Ice** is best in acute situations, such as a new injury or flare-up. It reduces inflammation by restricting blood flow and numbing pain. For best results:
  - Apply for **20 minutes**
  - Expect three stages: cold → aching → numbness
  - Remove the ice for **40 minutes**, then repeat if needed
- **Heat** should be reserved for chronic stiffness or muscle tightness—not fresh injuries. Heat increases blood flow, which can **worsen inflammation** if used too soon.

Doctor's advice: If you were in a car crash yesterday and apply heat today, you'll likely feel worse tomorrow. Use ice instead.

A hot shower or heating pad works well for old injuries or stiff areas.

Option C: Get some Over-the-Counter Medications

Many people reach for things like Tylenol, Advil, Ibuprofen, Motrin, or Aspirin. These non-steroidal anti-inflammatory drugs (NSAIDs) can provide short-term relief—**but you should only use them for a couple of days.**

Long-term use has consequences, including potential damage to your stomach lining and even **blocking the formation of new cartilage**, which your joints need to heal.

Option D: Go Visit Your Medical Doctor

This is often the first step people take, and your doctor may suggest one of three things:

1. Prescription Medications

These may ease symptoms temporarily—but consider this analogy:

If your house is on fire and your smoke alarm goes off, taking medication is like removing the battery. You didn't stop the fire—you just silenced the warning.

Sometimes, medication is necessary. I personally take prescription eye drops for glaucoma, which runs in my family's DNA. There's no alternative at this point. But medications can often come with side effects. For example, **Prednisone**, a common anti-inflammatory steroid, has an extensive list of potential effects including:

- Mood changes, insomnia, sudden weight gain, acne
- Weakened immune function
- Increased risk of osteoporosis

- Possible vision problems
- Decreased libido, fatigue, and weak muscles

And that's just scratching the surface. Take one medication for a side effect, and you may soon find yourself on two or three more.

Worse yet, many inflammatory problems start with poor diet—imbalances in Omega-3 vs. Omega-6 fats and too much processed or saturated fat feeding the inflammatory cycle.

2. Physical Therapy

You may be sent for PT, where you'll stretch and exercise. That's helpful in many cases—but often it's something you've probably already tried yourself.

3. Surgery

With so many other treatment options available surgery should be a last resort. If you are told surgery is needed I would get a 2nd opinion before committing!

According to Google:

- **1–4%** of patients die during surgery
- Up to **15%** have serious complications
- **5–15%** are re-admitted within 30 days

The riskiest surgeries include pancreatic, esophageal, and spinal procedures.

Maybe you'd rather go the non- medical route and try more conservative things like:

Yoga

Yoga can be great for increasing flexibility and easing tight muscles. If your issue is purely due to stiffness, this might help. But for deeper structural or neurological problems, it's usually not enough.

Massage

Massage feels amazing—and for good reason! It stimulates **mechanoreceptors** in your body that can override pain signals. It also promotes relaxation and helps move toxins out of the tissues (so drink plenty of water after).

However, massage doesn't diagnose the root of the problem, nor does it address **nutritional** deficiencies that could be contributing to chronic inflammation or pain.

Acupuncture

Acupuncture works by stimulating specific points on your body to rebalance your energy flow—known as "Chi"—and release natural endorphins.

Based on **Five Element Theory**, each element (Water, Wood, Fire, Earth, Metal) corresponds to specific organs and meridians:

- There are **12 major meridians**, named for organs like Lung, Liver, Kidney, etc.
- Emotions are also believed to affect health: for example, **Anger affects the Liver**, and **Worry impacts the Stomach**.

Acupuncture can be effective, especially when integrated with other forms of care.

Vitamins and Supplements

Vitamins are important—but how do you know which ones to take, and what brands to trust?

I personally use **NutriWest** in my practice. Founded by a Chiropractor in the 1982, they use high-quality ingredients and rigorously test for purity. They're based in Wyoming, and only available through healthcare professionals.

See a Chiropractor

Chiropractic is a specialty focused on your **nervous system**. Chiropractors don't prescribe drugs—that's what medical doctors do. But a good question to ask your Chiropractor is:

"How do you assess and improve nervous system function?" (You'd probably surprise them with such a well-educated question!)

A lot of Chiropractors rely on basic tools like:

- Motion palpation
- Leg length checks
- Surface EMG scans
- X-rays to show spinal distortion

While these tools aren't bad, they're a bit outdated. And too many doctors assume that school taught them everything they need to know, but the truth is:

The Real learning starts after school ends.

That's why it's called a **practice**—we're constantly practicing to improve our skills.

I believe there's a better way. We live in the 21st Century, and modern chiropractic care can incorporate advanced techniques, integrative nutrition, with individualized assessments.

A quote that comes to mind is *"When the student is ready, the teacher will appear."*

Doctors and patients could both be helped being open minded to new solutions—and willing to take the first step toward real healing. And that's what I want to teach you next, about an advanced method called Applied Kinesiology.

Applied Kinesiology: A Better Choice

In my opinion, the most effective and comprehensive method for analyzing the human body and uncovering what's really going on is called *Applied Kinesiology*—or muscle testing as applied to the human body.

Why?

Because it evaluates all three key aspects of health: physical, chemical, and emotional. It can identify structural issues that may be interfering with your body's optimal function, as well as nutritional remedies that may support your recovery.

It can also reveal underlying emotional factors that could be contributing to your condition. AK even allows us to assess the acupuncture system and pinpoint which meridians need support.

Using muscle testing, we can gain insight into the state of your digestive system, immune system, and endocrine system—each of which plays a critical role in how your body functions.

It helps uncover areas of distress receiving negative sensory input. In short, muscle testing gives us a functional "window" into what's happening inside your body.

It covers a lot of ground.

How does it work?
Muscle testing provides a basic yes-or-no response from the nervous system. A muscle either tests strong or weak. By applying different sensory inputs and observing how the muscle response changes, we're able to evaluate how the nervous system is reacting—remember: sensory in, motor out.

So what happens during a visit?
When new patients come in, it may or may not be their first visit to a chiropractor. But almost without exception, it *is* their first experience with muscle testing and Applied Kinesiology.

That's because AK is an advanced technique, and it's not typically part of the standard chiropractic curriculum. Chiropractic school focuses on preparing students to pass their board exams and get licensed—but the real learning begins in the "real world," working with real patients. And more often than not, the tools taught in school aren't enough to help people with complex issues.

Many doctors, once they're licensed, consider their education "good enough" and continue practicing based on what they learned in school. Sure, we're required to take a certain number of continuing education hours each year to maintain our licenses, but much of that material is just a rehash of what we already learned.

Because of this, after a new patient consultation, I often ask, "Have you ever been muscle tested before?" And most often, the answer is "no."

So before we begin, I offer a simple analogy to prepare the patient's mind:

"Imagine for a moment that you were born before the invention of the electric light bulb, and you're using candles or oil lamps to light your home at night. Then one day, someone shows you *this*."

At that point, I'll get up and manually turn the light switch off and on to control the overhead lights in my office.

I continue:

"What would you think?"

Most people respond with, "Wow!" or "That's magic!"

Right—but we know it's not magic. It's electricity. It's technology.

The same concept applies to muscle testing. You'll see weak muscles become strong again, and strong muscles become weak under the right conditions. But it's not *magic* or *voodoo*—it's *neurology*.

This approach allows the doctor and patient to communicate clearly throughout the exam. When patients see and feel what happens during muscle testing, they understand what's going on.

And if you want to dive deeper into how this works, read the chapter in Part 3 on *"The Neurology Behind Applied Kinesiology."*

A Detailed History to Bring the Doctor Up to Speed

Before we get into the muscle testing portion of the visit, it's essential to sit down and talk about why the patient is here and what they hope to achieve. Taking a thorough history gives the doctor insight into the problem and how it started. We want to know how long it's been going on, whether it's the first time or a recurrence, and how frequently it's happening now.

We also ask about any previous traumas—sports injuries, car accidents, falls, broken bones, surgeries, or anything else that might be relevant.

Next, we want to know what the patient has already tried to fix the issue. This helps us avoid wasting time on treatments that haven't worked.

We also ask how the problem feels—sharp, dull, burning, achy—because these descriptions can help us determine what's really going on. The severity of the pain matters, too. A "10 out of 10" pain with no obvious trauma might indicate something very different than a "10" following a car accident. In fact, the lack of a clear cause for extreme pain often means we need to look more closely.

It's also important to understand how this issue is interfering with daily life, and what the patient hopes to gain by resolving it. For example: "I want to get rid of these headaches so I can interact with my family again instead of spending the day in a dark room." When the doctor and patient are aligned on the goal, care becomes more focused and meaningful.

Finally, we ask: Is the condition getting worse, improving, or staying the same? That gives us a better sense of urgency and direction.

Once We Have the History, We Can Start Looking at the "Big Picture"

The body is a complex system, and before we zoom in on specific complaints, we start by stepping back and assessing the "big picture." Often, resolving a major underlying issue can naturally correct several smaller problems. By looking at overall patterns and imbalances first, we can be more efficient and effective in care.

Posture

A person's posture offers valuable clues about what's happening in their body. It's one of the smartest places to start when evaluating someone's physical condition. Postural imbalances often indicate chronic muscle weaknesses or compensation patterns from old injuries that may still be affecting the person today.

We start by observing the position of the hands. In a neutral stance, the thumbs should point forward with the palms facing the sides of the body. If the palms rotate backward and the thumbs point inwards, this often indicates weakness in the **teres minor**—a pattern we commonly see in patients with hypothyroid tendencies.

Next, check the **level of the shoulders**. Uneven shoulders may point to past trauma and should prompt an evaluation of the **upper trapezius** muscles.

Look at the **knees**—if they angle inward, it may indicate a weak **sartorius**, which can often correlate with **adrenal stress**.

Observe the **feet**. Are they pointing straight ahead? If one foot is rotated outward, consider evaluating the **psoas** or **gluteus maximus**.

Finally, assess whether the **hips are dropped** and if there's a **head tilt** to the same side. This combination can suggest a weak **gluteus medius**.

Range of Motion

Range of motion refers to how far and how well a body part can move through its normal path of motion.

There are two types of range of motion: **active** and **passive**.

- **Active range of motion** is how well you can move a joint using your own muscles.
- **Passive range of motion** is how far the joint can move when someone else moves it for you, without your muscles doing the work.

It's important to assess both types for several reasons. First, if there's a limitation in movement, testing both helps determine whether the restriction is due to muscle tension or an issue within the joint itself. Second, measuring range of motion gives us a baseline we can refer back to after treatment.

It helps answer the question: *"Does that feel better when you move it now?"*

Let's take the shoulder as an example. If you actively raise your arm and it hurts, we'll want to know: does it still hurt when you relax the arm and let the doctor move it for you? By taking the muscles out of the equation, passive range of motion helps us check the condition of the shoulder joint itself. This comparison helps us narrow down where the problem is actually coming from— whether it's the muscles, the joint, or both.

Another example is the neck. If you turn your head to look over your shoulder and the range of motion is only 60 degrees, but we know the normal minimum is 70 degrees, that tells us something's off. That's why we document not only the quality of active and passive motion, but also the measurable range—in degrees—so we have a clear, objective baseline to track progress over time.

Do Weak Muscles Respond Normally?

Let's say we find some weak muscles during the exam. The first thing we want to determine is *why* they're weak— and the priority is to rule out injury as the cause.

One way to do this is by stimulating the **muscle spindle**, located in the belly of the muscle. When you do this, one of two things will happen:

1. The muscle momentarily strengthens ("turns back on"), or
2. It remains weak.

What do these responses mean?

If the muscle *turns back on*, we know the weakness isn't due to an injury. Why? Because if there *were* an injury, it would override that temporary stimulation we just gave it. But if the muscle *remains weak*, it suggests there's an injury somewhere in the body that's neurologically inhibiting that muscle.

So how do we find where the injury is?

There are a few ways to do that. But first, let's put it in context.

Imagine someone trying to hammer a nail and they accidentally hit their thumb. What's the first thing they do after yelling in pain? They might rub it, shake their hand, or even put their thumb in their mouth.

Why do we instinctively do that?

Because rubbing or shaking the area stimulates **mechanoreceptors**—sensory receptors that send messages to the brain. These signals can temporarily override pain signals.

We use this bit of neurology to our advantage. When we gently rub the skin over an area of suspected injury, it can activate those mechanoreceptors, temporarily silencing the pain input that's shutting down the muscle. If the weak muscle suddenly turns on, we've likely found the site of injury—and now we know where to apply **Injury Recall Technique**.

Another method

Another way to locate old or hidden injuries is to have the patient touch the area themselves. Then, while they maintain contact, we extend the head and neck and retest a previously strong muscle. If that muscle weakens, the area they touched is likely connected to the problem. This also guides us to where Injury Recall Technique is needed.

Back to the muscle spindle

Now, let's circle back. If stimulating the muscle spindle briefly turned the muscle on, we know the issue isn't injury-related. However, that sensory effect only lasts about five seconds. When you test the muscle again, it'll usually go weak again—so we continue with additional tests to identify the real source of the dysfunction. We'll cover those next.

One More Thing About Weak Muscles

There's another layer to understanding weak muscles—one we haven't touched on yet: the **muscle-organ relationship**.

In some cases, a weak muscle may not only reflect a structural issue or past injury—it could also be connected to dysfunction in a related organ. These relationships are based on patterns of neurological and energetic connections in the body.

Here are some commonly observed muscle-organ correlations:

- **Pec Major Sternal** → Liver
- **Pec Major Clavicular** → Stomach
- **Tensor Fascia Lata** → Large Intestines
- **Psoas** → Kidneys
- **Sartorius & Gracilis** → Adrenal Glands
- **Quadriceps** → Small Intestines
- **Hamstrings** → Large Intestines
- **Gluteal Muscles** → Reproductive Organs
- **Biceps** → Stomach
- **Triceps** → Pancreas
- **Popliteus** → Gallbladder
- **Deltoids** → Lungs
- **Lower & Middle Trapezius** → Spleen
- **Infraspinatus** → Thymus Gland
- **Teres Minor** → Thyroid
- **Supraspinatus** → Brain & Nervous System

So, when we find a weak muscle, we don't just look at the joint or muscle itself—we also keep in mind that there may be a deeper, internal component at play.

That's why it's so important to evaluate the **systemic effects of old or hidden injuries first**. Once we've ruled those out or addressed them, we can start looking at broader patterns, including possible organ involvement.

Finding Old Injuries with Cerebellar Tests

The **cerebellum** is the part of the brain responsible for balance, coordination, and the unconscious control of posture. It's also where "muscle memory" of past injuries can be stored. That's why we use specific tests to assess cerebellar function when we suspect an unresolved or hidden injury.

Romberg's Test

One simple and effective test is called **Romberg's Test**. Here's how it's performed:

1. Have the patient stand with their feet together, shoes off.
2. Arms should be lifted to shoulder height and extended out to the sides—like forming a big letter "T."
3. Ask the patient to close their eyes and maintain that position.

If there's an old injury, the body will often sway or fall toward the **side of the dysfunction**.

Making It More Challenging

To increase the difficulty and sensitivity of the test, try these variations:

- **Single Leg Balance Test**: Have the patient stand on one leg with their eyes open. Difficulty maintaining balance on one side may point to an old injury on that side.

- **Single Leg with Eyes Closed**: Same test, but with the eyes closed. If balance fails or they fall to one side, it typically indicates that side is neurologically affected.

Why This Works

The cerebellum relies on **three major sources of input** to maintain balance:

- Visual information (eyes)
- Vestibular input (inner ear)
- Proprioception (feedback from the feet and body)

By removing visual input—i.e., closing the eyes—we stress the other two systems. If the cerebellum isn't processing proprioceptive or vestibular signals properly due to a past injury, balance will be compromised, and the body will compensate or collapse toward the weaker side.

These simple tests can help reveal old, unresolved injuries that may be affecting posture, coordination, or muscle function—even if the patient isn't consciously aware of them.

Deleting the Effects of Old Injuries with IRT (Injury Recall Technique)

So once we locate the site of an old injury, what do we actually do about it?

That's where **Injury Recall Technique**, or **IRT**, comes in.

IRT wasn't developed within the chiropractic profession—it was actually created by a podiatrist. The story goes that a chiropractor, seeking treatment for plantar fasciitis, visited this podiatrist and had the issue resolved using what we now know as IRT. Fortunately, that chiropractor saw the value and brought it into our field.

Interestingly, the key structure involved in this technique is the **talus bone** in the ankle—*the only bone in the body without a direct muscular attachment*. That uniqueness may be part of why it holds a special relationship with injury memory stored in the nervous system.

How IRT Works

Once an area of previous injury is located, here's the basic process:

1. **The patient touches the area** of suspected injury.
2. **The head and neck are placed in extension.**
   This combination seems to bring the injury memory to the surface neurologically.
3. Then, we apply a **gentle distraction to the talus bone**.
   This light contact is enough to "reset" the cerebellum's stored memory of the injury— essentially *deleting* the pattern from the nervous system.

For **injuries above the shoulders**, such as in the neck, we use a similar principle—but instead of the talus, we apply a **gentle flexion of the head on the atlas (C1)**. This may work because many neck injuries involve forced extension (e.g., in car accidents), and creating the opposite movement helps reset the system.

More Aggressive IRT (When Needed)

In some stubborn cases—especially in the neck—you may need to go a step further. Here's the modified approach:

- Apply pressure at both the **origin and insertion** of the affected muscle or ligament, pushing them together.

- This encourages the tissue to "reset" its stored memory.
- Then, follow with the **head flexion** as you would in standard IRT.

Advanced Neurological Confirmation: Eye Movement Testing

This next part is more advanced and might sound "out there," but for completeness, I'm including it.

Once you find the injury point using the standard IRT setup (patient touches the site, head extended, and a previously strong muscle now tests weak), you can confirm the **priority** of that injury by using the eyes.

Here's how:

- Without moving their head, have the patient **move their eyes toward the injury site**.
  - If the injury is **in front**, they should look **down** toward it.
  - If the injury is **on the back**, have them look **up**, as if trying to glance behind their head.
- Then, retest the previously weak muscle.

If it turns strong, you've confirmed the injury is **primary** and it should be treated directly with IRT.

If it doesn't strengthen, have them look in other directions.

- If a **different direction** causes the muscle to strengthen, this indicates the injury is **secondary** to a deeper issue—usually involving the **adrenal glands** or **parathyroid**.

In that case, you need to evaluate and treat those endocrine organs first. Once that's handled, retest the injury point. If it no longer weakens a strong muscle during the standard test, you've cleared it.

Rechecking After Treatment

One of the best parts about using muscle testing is the ability to **immediately reassess** after a treatment. If the injury truly was the root cause, muscles that previously *didn't* respond to stimulation (like a spindle stretch) will now **turn back on, even if still weak**. That's your confirmation the injury memory was cleared.

Just remember: if a muscle still tests weak after IRT, it may have other causes—nutritional, structural, or organ-related—but at least it's no longer neurologically inhibited by that old injury.

Acupuncture Pain Relief Techniques

At this point in the exam, if the patient is experiencing acute pain, we can pause and apply acupuncture-based pain relief techniques before continuing. There's no need to put someone through the full rigors of an exam when they're already in pain—we want to help, not aggravate.

In our office, we use two effective techniques that involve acupuncture points on the face:

1. **NSB (Nociception Stimulation Blocking)**
2. **Set Point Technique**

1. Nociception Stimulation Blocking (NSB)

NSB is used in acute situations—specifically when moving a body part causes pain. During this movement, we perform a muscle test. If the muscle weakens in response, that indicates nociceptive input (pain/stress signals) is interfering with proper function.

We then test acupuncture points on the face that correspond to the six meridians which either begin or end there. These "B&E" (Beginning & Ending) points include:

- **Large Intestine 20** – One of the most powerful points
- **Small Intestine 19**
- **Triple Heater 23**
- **Gall Bladder 1**
- **Stomach 1**
- **Bladder 1**
- Additional points to consider:
    - **Governing Vessel 26**
    - **Conception Vessel 23** (both located on the midline)

Here's how it works:

While the patient moves the painful area, you briefly tap each acupuncture point on the face, one at a time. After each tap, retest the previously weak muscle. If the muscle now tests strong, that's your spot. Tap that point approximately 100 times (or until the patient begins to feel relief).

It's a powerful, non-invasive way to quickly reduce acute pain—and I use it often with excellent results.

2. Set Point Technique

The Set Point technique is similar but is typically used for **chronic** pain or lingering injuries.

To find the right acupuncture point, have the patient touch the painful area. While they maintain contact, tap each of the facial acupuncture points as you muscle test. The correct point is the one that **weakens** the muscle in this case. That's your treatment point.

As with NSB, you then tap the point about 100 times.

This approach works by neurologically "resetting" the system and bringing relief to chronic patterns of dysfunction or pain.

These techniques are a great example of how Applied Kinesiology and acupuncture principles combine to provide fast, effective relief—especially when traditional methods fall short.

Checking for Inflammation with Aspirin and Benadryl

Remember how one of your treatment options was to try some over-the-counter medications? Well, we want to muscle test you first to see if that approach would actually work for you. If your muscle tests weak and it's *not* due to an injury, the next most common cause is **inflammation**.

Two Main Types of Inflammation

One type of inflammation is caused by an imbalance of dietary fatty acids. There are two key groups:

- **Omega-3 fatty acids** — found in fish oil, flaxseed oil, and walnut oil — are *anti-inflammatory*.
- **Omega-6 fatty acids** — found in sunflower, safflower, avocado, corn, soybean, and canola oils — can be *pro-inflammatory* when consumed in excess.

Too much Omega-6 can fuel inflammation by increasing prostaglandin production. That's why many people turn to over-the-counter medications like **aspirin**, **Tylenol**, or **Advil (NSAIDs)** to reduce inflammation.

We can use muscle testing to see if this type of inflammation is affecting you. If taking a small amount of aspirin (or another NSAID) temporarily strengthens a weak muscle, that's a strong clue that inflammation is the issue.

Next, we can test you with Omega-3 oil. For example, placing a drop of flaxseed oil on your tongue may immediately strengthen a weak muscle if fatty acid imbalance is the underlying cause.

What If it's Not Fatty Acid Inflammation?

If the muscle is still weak, we look at the next most common cause: **histamine-related inflammation** — often linked to allergies.

Histamine problems can happen for three reasons:

1. Your body is **producing too much histamine**.
2. You're **consuming too many histamine-rich foods**.
3. Your body **isn't breaking down histamine properly** due to nutritional issues.

Breaking down histamine efficiently requires **folic acid**, **vitamin B6**, and **vitamin C**.

To test this, we use **Benadryl**, an over-the-counter antihistamine. If Benadryl temporarily strengthens your weak muscle, it suggests a histamine issue — and that you may benefit from B6 and folate.

But What If You're Already Taking B6 and Folate?

You might be wondering why you'd still have histamine issues even if you're already taking a multivitamin. The answer lies in **vitamin activation**.

- **Vitamin B6** must be converted into its active form, **Pyridoxal-5-Phosphate (P5P)**.
- **Folic acid** must be converted into **methylfolate** to be properly used by the body.

Some people have genetic variants — such as **MTHFR mutations** — that reduce their ability to make these conversions.

That's why we can also muscle test you against **P5P** and **methylfolate** directly. If either one strengthens a weak muscle, your body likely needs that specific active form to function optimally.

Check Nutritional Status for Muscle Health
(Vitamin E, C, Iron, B12, Folic Acid, Cholesterol, Glucosamine & Chondroitin)

Now that we've ruled out other causes of muscle weakness, we can move on to assessing whether **nutritional deficiencies** are contributing to the issue.

Key Nutrients and What They Do

- **Vitamin E** is often helpful for **low back muscles**.
- **Vitamin C** tends to support **shoulder muscles and connective tissue**.
- **Vitamin B12** is critical for nerve and muscle function — especially important for **vegetarians**, since it's mostly found in animal products.
- **Iron** is essential for oxygen transport in muscles, particularly in **women of reproductive age**, who are more prone to deficiency.

- **Folic Acid** supports healthy red blood cell production and plays a role in methylation pathways (as we've discussed before).
- **Glucosamine and Chondroitin** are structural components of **joint cartilage**. If your body isn't making enough, supplementation may help — but we also want to ask *why* your body isn't producing them effectively in the first place.

Remember, our goal isn't just to cover up symptoms, but to uncover the **root cause** of dysfunction.

What About Cholesterol?

Cholesterol is a crucial part of cellular health and hormone production, but it needs to be properly metabolized. That's why we include a **muscle testing screen for cholesterol** and related liver function.

☐ Note: Muscle testing isn't a replacement for lab work, especially with cholesterol. It's more of a functional screen — something that can guide us toward what to test next.

Liver-Muscle Connection

The **liver** plays a major role in cholesterol metabolism. Here's something fascinating:
The skin over your liver and the liver itself share the same **neurological pathway** to the spinal cord. This means the brain can't tell whether stimulation is coming from the liver or the skin over it — we use that to our advantage.

When we **rub the skin** over the liver area, we stimulate the **parasympathetic system**, increasing liver function.

When we **pinch the skin**, we activate the **sympathetic system** (the "fight or flight" system)

Interpreting the Response

- If **rubbing** the liver area **strengthens a weak muscle**, we may suspect:
    - A **cholesterol processing issue**
    - Or **immune system involvement** (cytokines)
- If **pinching** the liver area **strengthens a weak muscle**, we may suspect:
    - **Liver toxicity (possibly an allergen as well)**
    - Or **triglyceride imbalance**

Either way, the next step would be to **confirm with lab testing**. But if we then test a targeted **nutritional support** in the office and it instantly improves muscle strength — that's a powerful validation of what the body needs.

One of these scenarios is likely to strengthen the weak muscle — and give us a real-time direction for supporting your health.

By the way, the skin over the liver is what we call a **Visceral Referred Pain** area (or "VRP") for the liver. There are multiple VRPs across the body that corresponds to different internal organs — and not all of them are located directly over the organ itself.

For example, the **spleen's VRP** is located over the *left shoulder*, near the deltoid muscle.

Checking for Free Radicals with the Bleach Sniff Test

Remember when we talked about **free radicals** — those unstable molecules that can damage your body and make you feel like you're 80, even if you're not? Well, we can actually check your body's ability to handle oxidative stress using a simple test: the **Bleach Sniff Test**.

What's the Connection?

Bleach contains **free radicals**, specifically in the form of **hypochlorite** — the same substance your **white blood cells** produce to destroy bacteria and viruses. When your immune system detects an invader, it fires hypochlorite at the cell, rupturing its membrane and killing it.

In this case, bleach acts as a stand-in for **oxidative stress** in the body.

How the Test Works

This is a simple **sensory-in, motor-out** test. Here's how we do it:

1. You sniff a sealed vial with a small amount of bleach (we don't want direct exposure — just enough to trigger a sensory input).
2. We then **muscle test a previously strong muscle**.

Interpretation:

- **If the muscle stays strong:**
  Your body is likely handling oxidative stress just fine — your antioxidant systems are keeping free radicals in check.

- **If the muscle weakens:**
  This suggests you may have **too many free radicals** circulating, overwhelming your system. Possible causes include:
    o **Autoimmune activity**
    o **Liver dysfunction**
    o **Heavy metal toxicity**
    o **Poor homocysteine metabolism**
    o **Environmental allergies or chemical sensitivities**

We'll use muscle testing to narrow down which of these may be the underlying issue.

- **If sniffing bleach makes a *weak* muscle become *strong*:**
  That's a red flag for a **low-functioning immune system** — your body may not be generating enough oxidative power to defend itself properly.

This quick test gives us valuable insight into your body's internal environment. From there, we can dive deeper with nutritional testing or lab work as needed.

Checking Ammonia and Aldehyde Toxicity with Muscle Testing

Your body naturally produces **ammonia** as a byproduct of **protein metabolism**. To safely process and move ammonia, it relies on liver enzymes such as **AST (SGOT)** and **ALT (SGPT)**. The **"T" stands for transaminase**, which requires **Vitamin B6** — specifically in its active form, **P-5-P (Pyridoxal-5-Phosphate)** — to function properly.

Ammonia Sniff Test

This simple test helps us determine how your body is managing ammonia levels:

1. You sniff a vial containing a small amount of **ammonia**.
2. We observe how your muscles respond through Applied Kinesiology.

Interpretation:

- **If ammonia weakens a strong muscle**:
  This could suggest:
  - **Elevated ammonia levels** already circulating in your body
  - **B6 (P5P) deficiency**
  - Possibly **kidney stress or dysfunction**

  Since B6 is also critical for making **brain neurotransmitters**, this test can also hint at deeper neurological or mood-related issues.

- **If ammonia strengthens a weak muscle**:
  This may indicate:
  - **Low protein intake** in the diet
  - **Poor protein digestion or absorption**

Aldehyde Sniff Test

Do you get headaches or feel nauseated from smells like **perfume, gasoline, cigarette smoke, or alcohol**? That may point to a **liver detoxification issue**.

Aldehydes are toxic byproducts of **alcohol metabolism**, and also of **yeast overgrowth** in the gut. These compounds are found in most artificial chemical smells.

We use **aftershave** for a quick aldehyde sniff test:

1. You sniff a vial of aftershave (a common source of aldehydes).
2. We check for muscle weakness.

Interpretation:

- **If the aftershave weakens a strong muscle**:
  Your liver may be struggling to clear aldehydes — possibly due to:
    - **Overburdened detox pathways**
    - **Yeast overgrowth**
    - **Chemical sensitivity**

  In this case, your body may benefit from **molybdenum**, a trace mineral that supports **Phase I and Phase II liver detoxification**, particularly in breaking down aldehydes.

These quick tests give us insight into how well your body is handling **metabolic waste and environmental toxins** — helping us decide whether nutritional support like **B6, protein, or molybdenum** might help restore balance.

Checking the Immune System with KI27, TMJ, and Cranial Indicators

As part of our assessment, we now move on to testing the **immune system**, which plays a central role in many hidden dysfunctions including headaches and vertigo.

KI-27 Acupuncture Point (Kidney 27)

This point, located at the junction of the **clavicle, first rib, and manubrium**, is highly sensitive and neurologically significant.

- **What we do**: You'll touch the KI-27 point while we retest a strong muscle.
- **What it tells us**:
    - If the muscle **weakens**, it strongly suggests a **cranial misalignment**.
    - The skull isn't a single bone — it's made of multiple plates, like a puzzle, that can shift or misalign due to stress, injury, or biochemical imbalances.

Interestingly, **80% of cranial faults** are **secondary to immune system problems**, not physical trauma.

TMJ (Temporomandibular Joint) Testing

Next, we evaluate the **TMJ** — the joint where your jaw meets your skull.

- **What we do**:
    - You'll touch both TMJs simultaneously.
    - Then we retest muscle strength, especially with your **head extended** (looking slightly upward).
- **What it tells us**:

71

- If this causes muscle **weakness**, it's often linked to an **injury pattern** tied to the immune system — again, in roughly 80% of cases.

We also look at **which side of the body** shows weakness:

- **Left-sided involvement** often correlates with **spleen stress**.
- **Right-sided involvement** may be linked to **thymus gland function**, which is crucial for making **T-cells** — the body's virus-fighting and anti-cancer immune cells (important in the context of things like COVID).

Lower Sternum and Chemical Sensitivities

- The **lower portion of the sternum** is another reflex point we check.
- Weakness here is often associated with **chemical sensitivities**.
- If this area is involved, we may **revisit the aftershave sniff test**, as aldehydes (toxic byproducts of chemical exposure) play a role.

Support tip: The trace mineral **molybdenum** is used by the **liver** to detoxify aldehydes.
A product we often recommend is **Total Alpha Lipoic Acid** by Nutri-West, which contains molybdenum.

Pre-Test Imaging: A Unique Phenomenon

Discovered by Dr. Wally Schmidt, this unusual finding came from a patient who had a **known weak muscle**. Yet, when retested, the muscle was **strong** — unexpectedly.

Dr. Schmidt asked what had changed. After some resistance, the patient finally admitted:

"If I think about the test before you do it, I stay strong."

This led to the concept of **Pre-Test Imaging**: the **mental act of anticipating a test** can temporarily override the dysfunction and show as strong.

This is especially relevant in **cranial misalignments**, as the **central nervous system** is involved in both motor control and intention.

We use this concept as another screening tool when evaluating complex immune and cranial interactions.

Checking the Citric Acid Cycle (Krebs Cycle)

The **Krebs cycle**, also called the **Citric Acid Cycle**, is one of your body's most important energy-producing systems. It happens inside your cells' mitochondria and is essential for making ATP — your body's energy currency.

Why It Matters

One of the major byproducts of the Krebs cycle is **carbon dioxide (CO_2)**. While most people think of CO_2 as just a waste gas, your body actually **needs it** for several key functions:

- **CO_2 + Water (H_2O) → (with Carbonic Anhydrase + Zinc) → Carbonic Acid**
- This Carbonic Acid breaks down into:
    - **Hydrogen ions** → used to make **Hydrochloric acid (HCl)** in your stomach
    - **Bicarbonate ions** → used by your **pancreas** to make digestive enzymes

So if the **Krebs cycle isn't working properly**, you may not make enough CO_2, which in turn affects digestion, energy, and overall metabolic health.

Why the Krebs Cycle Might Not Work

- **Inflammation**
- **Heavy metal toxicity**
- **Nutritional deficiencies** (like low Zinc or B vitamins)

The Paper Bag Test (Dr. Wally Schmidt's Method)

Here's the clinical trick:

- At this point in the evaluation, if we're still seeing a **muscle that stays weak**, and none of the prior steps have helped, we can check for a **Krebs cycle dysfunction** using the **paper bag test**.
- **What we do**:
    - You breathe gently into a paper bag for a short period — just like someone might do during hyperventilation.
    - This temporarily **increases your internal CO_2 levels**.
    -
- **What we're looking for**:
    - If that previously weak muscle suddenly becomes **strong**, it strongly suggests a **Krebs cycle issue** is affecting your energy metabolism.
    - We then know to explore:
        - Nutritional support for mitochondrial function (e.g., CoQ10, B-vitamins, Zinc, Magnesium)
        - Possible **heavy metal burden**
        - Detox or anti-inflammatory support if needed

This test usually comes up negative — but in those rare cases where it's positive, it can be a game-changer. You'd never know the Krebs cycle was the issue without this simple test.

Checking the Tonic Labyrinth Reflex (TLR)

The **Tonic Labyrinth Reflex**, or **TLR**, is one of the reflexes you were born with. It helps protect you from injury if you were to fall by coordinating certain muscle patterns — basically preparing your body to brace itself.

How TLR Works

Your body has two general types of muscles:

- **Flexors**: Bend joints (like your **biceps** or **hip flexors**)
- **Extensors**: Straighten joints (like your **triceps** or **quads**)

Here's how the reflex activates:

- When you're **lying down**, the body interprets that as potentially falling backward.
- In response, it **activates all the extensor muscles** and **inhibits the flexors** to brace for a fall.

Now, let's say you're lying down and **turn your head to the right**, simulating a fall to the right:

- Your body will activate the **right-side extensors** (like the triceps) and the **left-side flexors** (like the biceps and chest) to prepare for impact.

Using TLR in Muscle Testing

Let's say you've got a **weak left psoas** muscle. The psoas is a **flexor**.

- So, if we **turn your head to the right**, the **left-side flexors (including the psoas)** should automatically **turn on** due to the TLR.
- If this **doesn't happen** — and the left psoas stays weak — it tells us the TLR isn't functioning properly.

When this reflex doesn't do what it's supposed to, it's usually a sign that something **deeper is off**, most often in the **endocrine system** — especially the **adrenal glands**.

What We'll Do Next

If TLR fails to activate the correct muscle groups, our next step is to **evaluate adrenal function** and look more closely at the **endocrine system** to understand what might be disrupting your body's natural reflexes and energy balance.

Checking the Endocrine System

After evaluating the immune system, we move on to your **endocrine system**, which includes:

- **Adrenal glands** (stress response)
- **Thyroid gland** (metabolism)
- **Reproductive organs** (hormonal balance)
- **Pituitary and pineal glands** (master controllers in the brain)

The Hyper-Adrenal Challenge

Sometimes we encounter a patient who doesn't muscle test the way they should. For example, a muscle that *should be weak* stays strong. This usually indicates the person is in a **hyper-adrenal state** — in other words, their body is stuck in "go-go-go" mode.

These are often high-stress, Type A individuals who can't relax. Their system is running so hot that standard testing doesn't work as expected.

To evaluate this, we compare the **pituitary reflex** to the **adrenal reflex**:

- If stimulating both causes muscle weakness, that confirms **hyper-adrenal activity**.
- In this case, we identify an adrenal support supplement (often from NutriWest) to calm things down and restore accurate muscle testing.

☐ If no supplement works and testing remains abnormal, unfortunately, this person may **not be a good candidate for muscle testing**.

Adrenal Stress Test

If standard testing is functioning correctly, we move on to the **Adrenal Challenge**:

- We have the patient touch the **adrenal reflex point** (1 inch lateral and 2 inches up from the belly button) and test a strong muscle for weakening.

Ligament Stretch Test

- We can also apply a light stress to the **knee joint ligaments** and observe if a previously strong muscle weakens.

If this either of these occur, it likely means your adrenal glands are **overworked**. In that state, even minor physical stress is too much for your system to handle — which may mean **chiropractic adjustments should be delayed** until nutritional support is in place.

Chronic **ankle sprains** are a common sign of weak adrenals.

There's no one-size-fits-all adrenal supplement, but we often see benefits from **Vitamin C** and **B-complex vitamins**. We'll test to find what works best for your body.

Reproductive Gland Evaluation

To check reproductive health:

- We test the **gluteus medius muscle**, located on the outside of the hip.

- Weakness here may suggest **prostate issues in men** or **uterine dysfunction in women**.

Pituitary Gland Involvement

If *multiple endocrine muscles* are weak, the issue may lie with the **pituitary gland** (the "master gland") located at the base of the brain.

We use a method called **Pituitary Drive**:

- We evaluate **cranial bone movement** during breathing.
- If a deep breath (usually inhaling) improves strength, it indicates cranial tension is affecting pituitary function.
- We then apply gentle pressure to the skull during deep breathing to **restore cranial mobility** and **relieve pressure on the pituitary**.
- When done correctly, this often brings strength back to all endocrine-associated muscles.

Endocrine Cross Check

Sometimes multiple glands show signs of dysfunction. To determine which is the **priority**, we do an **Endocrine Cross Check**:

- We touch (therapy localize) various endocrine reflexes one at a time.
- The one that **turns on all the other weak muscles** is the one we need to address first.

Bonus Check: Liver & Pancreas

Since the **liver** helps detoxify hormones and the **pancreas** manages blood sugar, we do a quick screen here as well:

- **Rubbing the skin over the liver** mimics parasympathetic stimulation (rest-and-digest).
- **Pinching the liver area** mimics sympathetic stimulation (fight-or-flight).
- We observe how each affects your muscle strength to assess liver function.

This helps us better understand how well your body is handling its hormonal and metabolic workload.

Muscle Testing in Darkness – A Pineal Gland Check

This is a fascinating test because it simulates what's happening in your **endocrine system during sleep**.

The **pineal gland** is responsible for producing **melatonin**, the hormone that helps you fall asleep. Its activity is directly influenced by **light and darkness**:

- Light inhibits melatonin.
- Darkness stimulates melatonin production.

How the Test Works

We perform standard muscle testing under normal lighting conditions. Then we repeat the test **in the dark** (or with eyes closed/covered).

In a healthy system, muscle strength should be the same whether in light or dark.

However, if **multiple strong muscles suddenly weaken in darkness**, it strongly suggests **dysfunction in the pineal gland**.

Nutritional Support for the Pineal Gland

Once identified, we can test various nutritional supports to see what restores muscle strength in the dark. The most common options include:

- **Melatonin** (supports the hormone directly)
- **Potassium Iodide** (a key mineral for pineal function)
- **Nutriwest Pineal-Lyph** – a glandular supplement that includes support for pineal health

This test gives us a unique window into your **circadian rhythm**, **hormonal regulation**, and even **sleep quality** — all of which are closely tied to the pineal gland.

Checking the Digestive System

Next, we move on to evaluating the digestive system. This is an important part of your overall health, and muscle testing gives us a unique way to assess how well it's functioning.

We begin by checking for a **hiatal hernia** and evaluating the **diaphragm**, which is often involved when digestive issues are present.

Then, we assess the **ileocecal valve**—this is the connection between your small and large intestines, located on the right side of your abdomen. This valve can be either stuck open or closed, and both situations can cause problems. For example, excessive sugar intake is often linked to a valve that stays open, while undigested fats in the small intestine can cause the valve to remain closed.

On the opposite side of the abdomen (the left), we can also evaluate the **Houston valve**—which is essentially the internal anal sphincter. Dysfunction in this area can indicate issues in the lower digestive tract.

In addition to these core checkpoints, there are a few other reflex points I like to test:

- A point near the bony part of the pelvis on the **left side**, which can indicate the presence of **parasites**
- A point located **directly inside the belly button**, which can reveal a **yeast** imbalance

If testing any of these areas causes muscle weakness, we can then determine which **nutritional support** helps restore strength—giving us valuable information about what your body may need to correct the issue.

Checking the Emotional System

Next, we evaluate the emotional system. This step helps uncover whether unresolved stress or emotional patterns are affecting your body's function.

We begin by having you **place one hand across your forehead** and think about any stressful event or situation. Then we perform a muscle test. If your strength **weakens** during this process, it suggests your nervous system is reacting to that emotional stress.

To narrow things down, we'll have you **use your other hand** to touch specific areas—such as over your **liver** or **stomach**—while continuing to focus on that same emotional issue. If your muscle now tests **strong**, we've identified a related organ system, which in turn may correlate with a specific emotional pattern (e.g., liver often relates to anger, stomach to worry).

There's also an acupuncture point on the face—**Stomach 3**—that we can **tap while you're thinking about the issue**. This seems to help "break" the mind-body loop, or energetic imprint, of the stress. Many patients say they feel noticeably better after this technique. To confirm improvement, we'll retest you with your hand across the forehead to see if the muscle remains strong.

Sometimes more than one issue needs to be addressed— and that's okay. The beauty of this approach is that **you don't even have to say the issue out loud**. You simply think about it, and we evaluate your body's neurological response.

Emotional stress can also have a major impact on the **immune system**. That's why, when testing immune-related muscles, we'll often check to see whether an **emotional component** is involved. We do this by testing those weak muscles **against hypothalamus tissue**. The **hypothalamus** acts like a master switchboard, receiving and processing signals from all over the body—including emotional input. If the hypothalamus tissue doesn't affect the muscle response, we can rule out emotional stress as the source.

Once we complete this step, we've finished evaluating the **big picture** of what's affecting your health—physically, chemically, and emotionally.

Chapman's Reflexes

In the 1930s, osteopath Frank Chapman discovered reflex points on the body that appeared to correspond with specific organ dysfunctions. When these points were gently rubbed or stimulated, they often helped alleviate the symptoms patients were experiencing.

Later, it was found that these reflexes also influenced the function of certain muscles, deepening our understanding of the connection between muscles and organs, a concept central to Applied Kinesiology.

If a patient presents with weak muscles, we can now assess Chapman's reflexes to determine if stimulating these points has a positive effect on muscle strength. These reflex points are located at specific sites throughout the body. For a detailed map, you can search online for Chapman's Reflex locations.

Fascial Sheath

The next item to check during the exam is the *fascial sheath*. Normally, stretching a strong muscle should not cause it to weaken. If stretching *does* weaken the muscle, it indicates a need for fascial release.

This technique involves applying deep, sustained pressure along the muscle, almost like "ironing it out" to release tension or restriction in the fascia. After the release, re-test the muscle to see if stretching still causes weakness.

If this correction is needed repeatedly, it may suggest an underlying Vitamin B12 deficiency.

Iliolumbar Ligament in the Lower Back

One of the most common issues in lower back dysfunction involves the **iliolumbar ligament**. This ligament runs from the transverse processes of the fifth lumbar vertebra (L5) to the pelvis and can become strained due to faulty gait mechanics or repetitive stress.

To test for this issue, begin with a strong indicator muscle. Then apply a gentle pinch or pressure over the iliolumbar ligament area. If this weakens the previously strong muscle, it's a sign that the ligament may be involved.

The correction technique for this is known as **Injury Recall Technique (IRT)**. To apply it, contact both ends of the ligament and compress them gently toward the center of the ligament. Then, give a light "flick" to the **talus** bone in the ankle.

IRT was originally discovered by a podiatrist treating plantar fasciitis and was later adapted by Dr. Wally Schmidt, who recognized its broader application throughout the body. (Fun fact: the talus is the only bone in the body without any direct muscular attachments.)

When injuries occur, a reflex pattern is stored in the talus, acting almost like a "muscle memory" lodged in the cerebellum. The talus flick—done in a dorsiflexion direction—helps to "reset" or erase that memory, allowing normal function to return.

A similar reflex exists at the upper cervical spine, particularly involving the **skull and the atlas (C1)**. In cases of whiplash or hyperflexion/hyperextension injuries, this reflex can surface when the head is placed into extension. To clear it, gently flex the head forward onto C1 for a few seconds—this acts like a "delete button" for the neurological imprint of the injury.

Spine

With the patient lying face down, we can begin assessing for pelvic category problems. A **Category I** issue is identified by placing one hand on each sacroiliac (SI) joint and testing a previously strong indicator muscle. If the muscle weakens, it suggests a Category I pelvis— considered a *respiratory issue* within the pelvis and typically the least severe of the three pelvic categories. Fortunately, it's also the easiest to correct.

If the Category I test is negative, have the patient lift their head off the table. This allows you to evaluate the **neck extensor muscles**. Many neck problems actually originate from dysfunctions in the lower back, so this step helps identify those hidden links.

Next, ask the patient to turn their head to one side, then the other, while testing the strength of the neck extensors on each side. If weakness appears on one side, it often indicates an issue with the **pelvis on that same side**. To confirm, have the patient place a hand over the corresponding pelvic region—if the weak neck muscles strengthen, you've likely found the source of the problem.

From here, you can scan up the spine to check for **misalignments**. At each vertebral level, apply a light pinch or pressure and test your indicator muscle. If the muscle weakens, this suggests a subluxation—what chiropractors refer to as a misalignment that irritates the nervous system. That's your cue for where an adjustment may be needed.

Neck

Once the spine has been fully evaluated, we have the patient turn over to assess the neck. This process is called a **challenge**.

Start by identifying a strong indicator muscle—**Pectoralis Major Clavicular** is a convenient option since it's easily accessible in the supine position. Alternatively, the **psoas** can also be used, though it requires lifting the leg and testing at the feet.

To perform the neck challenge, turn the patient's head to one side while retesting the strength of your chosen muscle. Repeat on the other side. If turning the head in a particular direction causes the strong muscle to weaken, it suggests a misalignment that needs to be corrected **in that direction**.

After performing the cervical adjustment, re-challenge the neck by repeating the same head turn and muscle test. If the muscle remains strong this time, the correction was successful.

Pelvis

While the patient is still lying face up, have them therapy localize one sacroiliac (SI) joint at a time while you test a previously strong indicator muscle.
If the muscle weakens when they touch an SI joint, this suggests a **Category 2 pelvis** — often linked to **adrenal stress**.

A Category 2 means one side of the pelvis is out of alignment. At this point, check the muscles associated with adrenal function — especially the **Sartorius** and **Gracilis**. These muscles attach on the inside of the knee and run up toward the **pubic symphysis** and the **anterior superior iliac spine** (ASIS), the bony prominence on the front of the pelvis.

We often find related issues with the **foot on the same side** as the Category 2. So after correcting the pelvis, continue your assessment by working your way down the chain.

Feet

Next, we move down to the **feet** and perform what's called a **shock absorber test**. This involves using your fist to firmly tap the **balls of the feet**, the **arches**, and the **heels**, followed by a muscle test. If the muscle weakens, it suggests there may be **misalignments in the feet** affecting the body's structural balance.

If weakness is found, adjust the **feet, toes, arches, and ankles** as needed. Then repeat the shock absorber test. If the muscle now tests strong, the correction was successful.

Acupuncture System

Next, we assess the **acupuncture system**. In traditional Chinese medicine, acupuncturists perform what's called **pulse diagnosis**. There are **six pulses** on each wrist—**three superficial** and **three deep**—which correspond to the body's energy pathways.

We can integrate this system with **muscle testing**. If palpating a pulse causes a previously strong muscle to weaken, it suggests an energetic imbalance in that **acupuncture meridian**. From there, we can isolate the specific meridian involved.

Chinese acupuncture is built around the **Five Element Theory**—**Water**, **Wood**, **Fire**, **Earth**, and **Metal**. While *Fire* is technically a process, not a physical element, it's included due to its symbolic and energetic role.

You might ask, "Wait—five elements but six pulses?" Good question.

Here's how it breaks down:

- **Left wrist** (using the right hand's fingers):
    - Index finger: **Water**
    - Middle finger: **Wood**
    - Ring finger: **Fire**
- **Right wrist** (using the left hand's fingers):
    - Index finger: **Fire**
    - Middle finger: **Earth**
    - Ring finger: **Metal**

So, **Fire** is represented **twice**, covering four meridians total.

Each **element** is associated with specific **organs** and **meridians**:

- **Water**: Kidney, Bladder
- **Wood**: Liver, Gallbladder
- **Fire**: Heart, Small Intestine, Triple Heater (which governs respiration, digestion, and genitourinary function), and Pericardium (also called Circulation Sex, which relates to hormonal balance)
- **Earth**: Stomach, Spleen
- **Metal**: Lung, Large Intestine

Every **muscle in the body** corresponds to an acupuncture meridian. So, if you detect a weak pulse that correlates with a specific meridian, you'll often find a **related muscle** testing weak as well.

To confirm, you can **therapy localize** the meridian's **alarm point**—if a strong muscle goes weak during this, it verifies the issue. Treatment involves stimulating the **tonification point** to restore energy and function to that meridian.

Acupuncture is ultimately about **balance**.

"Ah yes, Daniel-san, you need balance!" — *Mr. Miyagi*

Anything Else?

At this point, we're almost finished. A quick **gait analysis** can help us catch any final imbalances we may have missed. Then, have the patient stand up and **recheck all the ranges of motion** that were previously painful. In most cases, they'll feel significantly better.

However, if the patient is **still experiencing pain**, especially in long-standing or chronic cases, we can turn to additional **acupuncture-based techniques**.

One of the most useful is called **LQM**, which stands for **Location, Quality, and Memory**.

When someone has been dealing with a problem for a long time, it can become **embedded into the nervous system**—almost like it becomes part of their identity. Keep in mind, the nervous system operates on a simple principle: **sensory in, motor out**.

Here's how LQM works:

1. **Location**:
   - Start with a strong muscle test.
   - Ask the patient to **think about the exact location of their pain**.
   - If the muscle now weakens, it shows a **sensory input** is causing a motor output weakness—indicating that the nervous system has internalized the pain.

   Next, tap on a set of acupuncture points around the face to find which one negates the weakness. The points to try are:

   - **LI20**
   - **SI19**
   - **TH23**

- ST1
- GB1
- BL1

Once the correct point is found, **stimulate it with tapping**—at least **100 repetitions** or until the pain improves. Re-test by having the patient think of the pain location again.

2. **Quality**:
   - Now ask, "What does the pain feel like?" (sharp, dull, burning, etc.).
   - Repeat the same procedure: test a strong muscle, have them focus on the **quality**, and tap the appropriate facial acupuncture point to correct it.
3. **Memory**:
   - Finally, ask them to recall **when the pain first started**.
   - Again, test for weakness and treat it the same way if it shows up.

This **LQM technique** is especially effective for **chronic pain patterns** that have gotten "stuck" in the nervous system.

There's one more tool you can use: the **Tonification Point Technique**.

- Begin by **testing acupuncture alarm points** along with a muscle test.
- If any of the points cause a strong muscle to weaken, have the patient **touch that alarm point** while you **stimulate the tonification point** associated with it—again, using about **100 taps**.
- This can restore proper energy flow through that meridian and help resolve lingering pain.

Gait Analysis

Dr. George Goodheart observed that when a patient's problem keeps coming back, it's often related to the way they walk—their **gait**.

Proper gait requires **certain muscles to be "on"** (firing correctly) while **others are "off"** (inhibiting at the right time). This coordinated pattern allows the body to move efficiently and pain-free.

In a normal walking motion, **your arms should swing opposite to your legs**—left arm with right leg, right arm with left leg. But if you take a moment to observe people walking in public, you'll be surprised how many have lost that natural rhythm. Many walk **without any arm swing at all**, a clear sign that their gait mechanics are off.

Poor gait leads to compensation patterns throughout the body, and these can **undo much of the work you've just done**. That's why evaluating and correcting gait patterns can be a critical final step in helping patients hold their adjustments and stay pain-free.

X-rays

Sometimes, taking **X-rays** is essential to understand what's going on with the spine and joints—especially when a patient has a neck injury, like whiplash. Not only do X-rays help document the injury for **medicolegal** reasons, but they also give us critical information for creating an effective treatment plan to help the patient return to "normal."

The primary things we're looking for on a neck X-ray are:

- The **spinal curves**—we need to check that they're present and properly aligned.

- The **disc and joint spaces**—we want to ensure these spaces are open and healthy.

Why is the neck curve so important?
In the office, I like to use a **"show and tell"** method to explain it. Let me walk you through it:

I use an **8-pound bowling ball** to demonstrate how much the head weighs.
I'll say to the patient, "Let's pretend this arm is your neck. Your head weighs about 8 to 10 pounds—just like this bowling ball. Now, I want you to hold the ball with your fingers in it, like this," (showing the wrist in a supported position, arm bent, simulating the curve of the neck).

"See how easy that is? But now, let's pretend you lose that curve in your neck." (I move the ball so the wrist straightens out.)
"Do you see how much harder that is? And after a while, that's going to start causing pain, right?"

"That's why it's important to maintain that curve in your neck. It helps support the weight of your head properly. Does that make sense?"

This simple visual helps patients understand the critical role that a healthy neck curve plays in supporting the head and preventing strain or injury.

Blood Work

Blood work adds an extra layer to our diagnosis, allowing us to **"see"** what's going on with your blood chemistry.

While many people are familiar with cholesterol and Hemoglobin A1C levels, there are other important factors to consider—such as the **size of your red blood cells**. As red blood cells mature, they are supposed to shrink in size. However, nutritional deficiencies, particularly in **B12** or **Folic acid**, can cause red blood cells to remain **larger than normal**. This abnormality can be detected in a standard **Complete Blood Count (CBC)**.

By assessing these levels, we can gain deeper insight into your overall health and tailor a more specific treatment plan.

DNA Analysis

As discussed earlier, DNA analysis is a fascinating way to examine our health by looking at **mutations** or **SNPs** (Single Nucleotide Polymorphisms) in the genes that are important for various bodily functions.

Your **genes** contain the instructions needed to produce the enzymes that regulate your body chemistry, and everything in this process is based on **organic chemistry** (yes, that dreaded college course!).

There are certain areas we prioritize when examining DNA to understand how well your body is functioning. One of the most critical processes we look at is **methylation**. Methylation involves moving a carbon molecule with three attached hydrogens from one substance to another. It plays a crucial role because it has the ability to **"turn off" bad genes** and **"turn on" good genes**. For example, many people are familiar with the **MTHFR** gene, which stands for **methylenetetrahydrofolate reductase** (now you can see why we use abbreviations!). This gene is a key player in methylation, and its status shows up in your DNA analysis.

Here are some other key areas we examine during DNA analysis:

1. **Brain neurotransmitters**: How well are they being produced and metabolized? Genes like **COMT** (Catechol-O-Methyltransferase) and **MAO** (Monoamine Oxidase) are important for brain function and mood regulation.
2. **Intestinal health and gluten tolerance**: We check the **HLA-DQ2.2** gene for gluten sensitivity, which plays a role in autoimmune conditions like celiac disease.
3. **Inflammation and histamine tolerance**: We assess **DAO** (Diamine Oxidase) and **HNMT** (Histamine N-methyltransferase) genes, which are involved in histamine breakdown and inflammation regulation.
4. **Mitochondrial health**: We look at **NDUF** genes to understand how well your cells are producing energy.
5. **Detoxification**: The **CBS pathway** genes are key to detox processes, helping your body manage toxins effectively.
6. **Cardiovascular health**: We analyze **NOS3** (Nitric Oxide Synthase) and other lipid-related genes to evaluate cardiovascular health and risk.
7. **Neurological health**: The **APOE** gene is linked to Alzheimer's risk and brain function, and we assess it to understand your neurological health better.
8. **Sulfur tolerance**: We look at **Glutathione** markers, as glutathione is one of the most powerful antioxidants in your body. It's made up of three amino acids: cysteine, glutamate, and glycine. Cysteine is where sulfur is found, which connects

to **Homocysteine** and **Methionine**, originating from the proteins you consume.

9. **Longevity markers**: One key marker is **CETP** (Cholesteryl Ester Transfer Protein), which has been linked to longer lifespan in certain genetic variants (e.g., the 'GG' and 'AA' variants). (10)

10. **Sleep**: Your DNA can also reveal insights into how well you sleep. To produce **melatonin**, your body must convert **Tryptophan** into **serotonin**, which then undergoes two enzyme reactions to form melatonin. If there are issues in this process, we can test various nutritional supplements like **P5P**, **B5**, or even **melatonin** itself to help improve your sleep quality.

Denneroll and Neck Rehabilitation

As we discussed in the X ray section, when people are involved in a car crash, they often suffer from what's called **whiplash**. But what exactly is a whiplash injury?

Your neck is designed to move in specific directions, but one at a time: forward, backward, turning right or left, and side-bending left or right. However, in a car collision, studies using high-speed cameras have shown that the neck can move in **two different directions at once**, which is not ideal. This type of movement places extreme stress on the ligaments in the neck that hold the bones together, often leading to injury.

The result is typically the **loss of the normal cervical curve**, which is designed to support the weight of your head. This same process can also happen gradually over time due to poor posture, especially for people who work long hours in front of computers (8 hours or more each day).

A rehabilitation device called the **Denneroll**, invented by a chiropractor in Australia, attempts to restore the normal curve in the neck using gravity. The device works by supporting your neck while you lie on it. Over time, with consistent use, the Denneroll can help improve the neck's curve.

The process is gradual—realistically, it can take up to **a year** to regain the proper curve, depending on various factors like disc degeneration or arthritis. The device is typically used for **20 minutes a day**, with users working their way up to that maximum time.

It's important to note that individuals who are less physically fit may find it more challenging to restore their neck's curvature. Rehabilitation is not a quick fix, but with consistent effort, many people experience significant improvement.

So, What Do I do now?

By now, you should have a clearer understanding of why you might be feeling like you're 80 years old and what you can do about it. Identifying the root cause of your discomfort is the first crucial step in regaining control over how your body handles the everyday stresses of life. This way, you can pursue your dreams and live the life you've always hoped for.

If you're ready to uncover what's going on with your body, it makes sense to seek out a practitioner who can address all the topics we've discussed. A doctor trained in Applied Kinesiology can be a great partner on your journey to feeling better and getting back to your best self.

Also, if you're interested in exploring DNA analysis to dive deeper into your health, it's easier and more affordable than ever. Simply order a test kit from Ancestry.com (typically around $99, and sometimes on sale during holidays). The kit includes saliva collection instructions, and once you return it, your results will be ready in about 8 weeks. You'll then be able to download your raw data, which we can analyze using our Functional Health Evaluation software to gain valuable insights tailored to your health.

Are you ready to take the next step?

If you're ready to start your journey toward better health, I'd love to help you get there. Since you read this entire book you're now entitled to receive a complementary one on one consultation and evaluation with me.

We will cover all the topics that were discussed here.

Feel free to reach out to me at **(303) 377-1755** to set up your time slot or to ask any questions you might have.

My office is located at **3333 South Bannock St #235, Englewood, CO 80110** in the old Wells Fargo Bank building.

Or for even more information or to book online, visit my website: **www.youneedmeback.com**.

Let's work together to help you feel and be your best!

I'd like to share with you now what other people have said about the work I do on the following pages.

Patient Testimonials (from Google)

Elizabeth Wallace

Dr. Ebeling is more than just a chiropractor. He's better than any chiropractor I've been to and better than any doctor I've seen. After 1 visit, I was already bragging about him to my husband and friends. I came in with intense pain in my upper back and neck. In the first visit he figured out the cause through his very thorough exam. The next day my back was instantly better! He/we found out that I was allergic to mold. And I truly believe it was by his technique that we figured this out. And I can tell you no normal doctor or chiropractor would have figured that out, especially after 1 visit! He's very informative on his work and methods. He addressed my other concerns with no problem. He also discovered more underlying health issues. I promise you will not be disappointed with Dr. Ebeling!

Delaney Dennis

Dr. Ebeling is the best of the best. I was having major vertigo that was going unsolved for almost a year. I had gone to multiple urgent cares & ERs who all couldn't figure out what was going on with me. I was extremely discouraged until I found Dr. Ebeling, the very first day I went to see him he had pinpointed the cause of my vertigo almost immediately & now I feel the best I've felt in a long time. I HIGHLY recommend Dr. Ebeling, he is the absolute best!

Alan Li

Dr. Ebeling is not your typical chiropractor who simply cracks and adjusts. His practice is unique, utilizing applied physiology and integrating structural, nutritional, emotional , and energy adjustments to achieve the best balance for your body.

I initially sought his help due to severe back pain. After just 2 adjustments, my back pain began to ease significantly. With consistent treatment over the next two to three months, I gradually regained the ability to exercise. A year later, my sleep quality has improved, I've resumed strength training, and by the end of this year, I even returned to the slopes for skiing.

I am incredibly grateful to Dr. Ebeling for helping me reclaim not just my physical health but also the active lifestyle I love!

Cameron Mascoll

I highly recommend Dr. Ebeling to anyone dealing with back pain, especially those who are skeptical about chiropractic care. After struggling with pain for years, I saw remarkable improvement in just two sessions with him. His approach changed my perspective, and would encourage anyone to give it a try, even if they're a doubter like I was.

Maria Mota

Since I started with Dr. Ebeling I noticed a lot of changes on my overall health. I feel stronger and healthier. I always thought I have good nutrition until I meet him. He reads your body and explains everything in detail to you. He is excellent! Please give him a try for a healthier you.

Jaime Salek

Highly recommend Dr. Ebeling! Cannot believe how far my back issue has come in just a few treatments! I was in so much pain and was afraid to get an adjustment, but Dr. Ebeling's methods are gentle and his thoughtful approach is refreshing.

Greg Aden

Robert provides peace of mind when I am in his care. He knows what to try to uncover the reason for the pain. He explains things in a way that allows me to understand the why. He's been great for me over the six plus months I've been seeing him.

Sabrina Adair

Dr. Ebeling's chiropractic work is pure magic! I have seen several different doctors over the course of a decade, and his services are hands down the best! Even as soon as a single session, the pain in my body is relieved, and I feel more in alignment! Highly recommend!

Dr. Lynn Toohey

Dr. Ebeling is an awesome chiropractor; his knowledge of advanced kinesiology never ceases to amaze me as he finds muscle weakness patterns and corrects imbalances. Dr. Ebeling was able to correct my neck where it had been previously resistant to chiropractic adjustment, and thoroughly explained why my neck needs a different approach. I would highly recommend seeing him for any issues you may have.

_____

And to see over 300 more reviews just like that look me up on Google.

Part 3

The History of Applied Kinesiology

In case you're interested, I decided to include a brief history of Applied Kinesiology—because I find it fascinating, and you might too.

In 1939, George Goodheart Jr., the future developer of Applied Kinesiology, graduated from the National College of Chiropractic in Lombard, Illinois, a suburb of Chicago. He joined his father, George Goodheart Sr.—also a chiropractor—in practice.

At first, George Jr. practiced traditional chiropractic care, but he felt there had to be more. After about 25 years in practice, someone gave him a book about muscle testing. He began using these techniques on his patients and found he could help many of them by manually manipulating weak muscles to make them strong again. One of his first successful cases using this method involved a shoulder problem, which he resolved by working on the origin and insertion of the weakened muscle he had identified.

Using muscle testing, he made numerous discoveries about how the body truly functions. He became so skilled—better than anyone else at the time—that in 1980 he became the **first chiropractor ever** asked to serve as a team doctor for the U.S. Olympic Team.

George practiced in Detroit, Michigan, and his next-door neighbors had two boys. Every so often, the neighborhood would get together for flag football. One day, one of the boys injured his wrist. George said, "Come here, I'll fix that for you!" The kid was amazed: "Oh my God, how did you do that?!" That moment inspired both boys to eventually become chiropractors.

One of those boys—nicknamed "Wally"—later became my teacher.

Wally was a genius in his own right. After graduating from Chiropractic College, he went on to earn an advanced degree in neurology. He could explain, in intricate detail, how and why chiropractic worked through the neurological pathways.

He worked in George's office for five years, soaking up everything George had discovered about muscle testing. Then, after three decades in private practice, he refined those teachings and organized them into a logical system that maximized patient outcomes. Eventually, he began teaching this system—and I was lucky enough to be one of his students.

Therapy Localization

Remember earlier when I mentioned that the nervous system has two primary functions—"sensory in" and "motor out"? We can use that basic idea to help identify areas of dysfunction in the body.

Here's how: When I test a strong muscle "in the clear" (meaning no extra sensory input is added), I can then introduce a new stimulus—like the patient simply touching an area of their own body—to see how that input affects the strength of the muscle.

I remember watching a YouTube video of Dr. Goodheart explaining how he discovered this technique, which he later called *Therapy Localization*, back in 1973. Here's the story:

A tennis player came in with carpal tunnel symptoms. George explained how misaligned carpal bones could put pressure on the median nerve, leading to hand weakness and difficulty gripping a racket. He had the patient hold her thumb and pinky together while he tested their strength. They were weak.

Then he instructed her to squeeze the bones of the forearm—specifically the radius and ulna—near the wrist while he retested the muscle. The idea was that this pressure might shift the wrist bones enough to temporarily relieve nerve compression. On the retest, the muscles were strong.

But the patient asked, "How did it get strong just from me *touching* it?"

Wait, what?

George had told her to squeeze the wrist bones, but apparently, she had just lightly *touched* the area. Odd. But he made a mental note.

A Tragic Turn and a Powerful Realization

Part two of the story is more somber. George's wife drank tomato juice from the refrigerator that had a broken seal. She contracted botulism, underwent abdominal surgery, and although she survived the procedure, she passed away from subsequent complications.

After the funeral, George sat in his study, grieving and reflecting. "How could this have happened?" he asked aloud. "We did blood work and X-rays, but we missed it!"

Then, as he told it on video, he heard a voice say:
"Because you're asking the wrong person."

Startled, he replied, "Well, who are you supposed to ask besides the doctor or the patient, whoever you are?"

The voice answered:
"You have to ask the patient to ask the patient."

That's when it clicked.

He remembered the tennis player and the moment her muscle strength improved just from touching the wrist. "Oh!" he realized. "When I have the patient touch an area and do a muscle test, I'm asking the patient to ask the patient."

That was 1973—and it marked one of the most important breakthroughs in understanding how to diagnose and treat human health issues using the body's own sensory feedback.

The Neurology Behind It

So that's how it works, neurologically speaking:

Mechanoreceptors are sensory receptors located all over the skin. Their nerve fibers travel to the spinal cord. Pain signals also travel via nerves and often arrive at the same spinal cord segments as those mechanoreceptor signals.

This overlap means that when mechanoreceptors are stimulated, they can temporarily override pain signals being sent to the brain.

That's why, back in the day, you'd see older folks rocking in chairs on the front porch. The repetitive motion stimulated mechanoreceptors, which in turn helped dull the pain of arthritis.

It's also the same principle behind a TENS unit (Transcutaneous Electrical Nerve Stimulation). These devices send mild electrical currents through electrodes stuck to the skin. The stimulation activates mechanoreceptors and muscle contractions, which override pain signals.

Think about the last time you hit your thumb with a hammer. After shouting "Ow!", (and maybe a few other words), what did you instinctively do? You rubbed it, shook it, or put it in your mouth. Why? Because you were now stimulating mechanoreceptors in the skin to block the pain.

This is also why a good massage "feels good" —you're activating those same receptors and interrupting pain signals.

So even if this concept of sensory override is new in theory, you've definitely seen it in action.

Putting It All Together

In the case of the tennis player, when she touched her wrist, it provided enough sensory input to stimulate her mechanoreceptors. That input temporarily overrode the carpal tunnel pain and allowed her muscles to function more normally. That's the essence of therapy localization—and one of the many ways Applied Kinesiology helps us "ask the body" for answers.

The Neurology Behind Applied Kinesiology and Injuries

Injuries and the Cerebellum

The **cerebellum**—that part of your brain located at the lower back of your skull—is responsible for the unconscious control of your **posture, balance, and coordination**. It constantly receives sensory information from all over the body and, as we discussed earlier, it decides how to respond to that information, primarily by adjusting muscle tone and contraction.

Now here's something truly fascinating: Injuries—no matter how old—can leave a lasting imprint on your nervous system.

The cerebellum doesn't just process sensory input in the moment. It also stores what we might call a "muscle memory" of past injuries. And unless something is done to actively **clear or reset** that pattern, the cerebellum will **hold onto that injury memory indefinitely**.

When I say "forever," I mean **for-e-ver**.

That means if you broke your arm when you were five and it healed completely, the cerebellum may still be holding onto that injury pattern—continuing to influence how the muscles around that arm fire or respond, even decades later.

What Counts as an "Injury"?

In Applied Kinesiology, we consider any negative input to the nervous system an "injury." It's not just broken bones or obvious trauma. Anything that causes **pain**, **stress**, or **disruption** to the body's communication system can leave a lasting neurological impression.

Here are a few examples:

- Broken bones
- Ankle sprains
- Root canals
- Surgeries (including any procedure done under anesthesia)
- Cuts, scars, and burns
- Mammograms
- Auto accidents
- Sports injuries
- Significant emotional or mental trauma

Some of these may seem minor—or long forgotten— but your nervous system may still be reacting to them, subtly affecting posture, strength, or coordination.

That's where Applied Kinesiology shines: by using muscle testing and other techniques, we can uncover these hidden injury patterns and work to clear them, helping restore proper neurological communication and function.

How Do We Know Someone Has Old Injuries Affecting Their Nervous System?

There are a number of ways to figure this out. The simplest? Just **look at their posture**.

As we discussed earlier, the **cerebellum** is responsible for the **unconscious control of posture**. So if you see someone standing with **uneven shoulders, a tilted pelvis, or a head that chronically leans to one side**, odds are there's an **old injury pattern** stored somewhere in their nervous system.

But posture is just the beginning.

A More Accurate Method: Therapy Localization

This is where **muscle testing** comes in. It allows us to interact directly with the nervous system. And this brings up an important point:

Chiropractors don't just work on backs—we work on **nerves**.

When I perform muscle testing, I'm evaluating the **motor output** of the nervous system. If a muscle that *should* be strong tests weak, it's usually not a muscle problem. It's a **nerve signal issue**—and that tells me there's a problem somewhere in the **sensory input** loop. My job is to figure out where that bad signal is coming from.

One way to do this is by starting with a known **strong muscle**, and then having the patient **touch an area** of their body—like an old injury, scar, or painful spot. If that muscle suddenly weakens, it tells us that part of the body is sending a **negative sensory signal**. That's **therapy localization**, and it's one of the cornerstones of Applied Kinesiology.

Receptors: The Locks and Keys of the Nervous System

To understand how all of this works, we have to talk about **receptors**. These are specialized nerve endings that detect changes in your environment and send that information to your brain.

Here's a simple analogy:

Think of a receptor like the **lock on your front door**. It only works if the right **key** (stimulus) is inserted.

Your body has millions of these receptors, and some of the most important ones for what we do are called **mechanoreceptors**—which respond to physical stimuli like **touch, pressure, vibration, movement, temperature, and even sound**.

Two Special Receptors in Your Muscles

There are two mechanoreceptors inside your muscles that are especially important for Applied Kinesiology:

1. The Muscle Spindle

Located in the **belly of the muscle**, this receptor responds to **stretch** by causing the muscle to **contract**. It helps maintain balance and posture and gives your brain a constant stream of information about where your body is in space. This is called **proprioception**.

In AK, we use this to test for imbalances. If we find a weak muscle, we can gently **stretch the belly** of the muscle (by separating the fibers slightly). If the muscle gets stronger for about **5 seconds**, it confirms the muscle spindle is functioning and the muscle is neurologically responsive.

2. The Golgi Tendon Organ (GTO)

Located where the muscle meets the tendon, the GTO does the **opposite** of the muscle spindle. When it senses a strong contraction, it briefly shuts the muscle down to prevent injury—like a circuit breaker tripping to stop an overload.

In testing, if you gently **pinch the ends** of a muscle together (mimicking contraction), the muscle should **weaken briefly** for about 5 seconds before returning to normal. This tells us the muscle is acting as a good **indicator muscle**—one we can trust in further testing.

What If Nothing Tests Weak?

Every once in a while, we come across someone who tests perfectly—**no weak muscles**, even when there *should* be.

Even the GTO stimulation doesn't produce the expected momentary weakness.

What's going on?

These people are usually stuck in a **hyperadrenal** state. Their nervous system is running so hot that it can't even **relax long enough to reveal a problem**. Maybe they're a high-stress personality (Type A), maybe it's mental/emotional stress, or maybe they're physically overloaded—but the system is in **survival mode**.

Before we can use AK effectively, we need to **calm the adrenals down**.

Resetting the System

To do this, I have them **therapy localize** the **pituitary point** (right between the eyebrows), while at the same time rubbing their **adrenal reflex points** (just above the kidneys on the back). If this causes a strong muscle to weaken, it confirms adrenal involvement.

From there, we test various **adrenal support supplements** to see which one helps. The right one will stop that weakness from happening again. After chewing the supplement, the patient should now test normally and be ready for further evaluation.

About the Author

I became a Chiropractor because of my mom.

When I was about 16 years old, she started having neck pain. She called her cousin—who happened to be a Chiropractor in another state—and he told her to find someone local. She did. But when she came back from her appointment, I could *see* it in her face—**she looked worse, not better**.

And I remember thinking, *"WTF? I thought she was supposed to feel better—what happened? I could probably do a better job myself!"*

So I did what I could. I started rubbing her shoulders and neck, moving her head around gently, just trying to help. She turned to me and said,

"You've got great hands—you should become a Chiropractor!"

And I said, "Okay, Mom!"

That moment changed my life.

I went on to earn a Bachelor of Science degree in Biology back in New Jersey, then attended the Los Angeles College of Chiropractic, where I graduated in 1989 on the **Dean's List**. A year later, I moved to Colorado and have been in private practice ever since.

I started my practice at age 27 thinking I knew everything—**because hey, I was on the Dean's List!** But I quickly realized: **I didn't know nearly enough.**

That realization drove me to learn more. Patients were coming in with issues I didn't know how to fix. I felt like something was missing. Then, about 10 years into practice, I enrolled in a yearlong intensive study of Applied Kinesiology with Dr. Robert Blaich, DC.

That program opened my eyes to how the body really works.

And just when I thought *now* I finally knew everything, I met **Dr. Wally Schmidt**—and he absolutely blew my mind. He showed me how to use muscle testing as a window into the **nervous system**. That changed everything.

These days, I'm humble enough to know that even though I've learned a lot, there's **always more to learn**. I like to think of it this way:

- **Dr. George Goodheart** was the teacher of
- **Dr. Wally Schmidt**, who became the teacher of
- **Me**.

So when you come see me, you're getting the benefit of **three generations of Applied Kinesiology wisdom**—passed down, refined, and ready to help you heal.

References

(1) https://medlineplus.gov/ehttps://www.hopkinsmedicin e.org/health/conditions-and-diseases/chronic-fatigue-syndrome#:~:text=Causes%20of%20Myalgic%20Enceph alomyelitis/Chronic,and%2C%20occasionally%2C%20re current%20infections.

(2) https://www.cdc.gov/me-cfs/about/index.html#:~:text=People%20with%20ME/C FS%20are%20not%20able%20to%20function%20the,he alth%20history%20and%20current%20illness.

(3) https://www.cdc.gov/me-cfs/causes/index.html#:~:text=Possible%20causes.%20 Because%20the%20cause%20of%20ME/CFS,infection% 2C%20inflammation%2C%20toxins%20or%20injury%2C %20and%20genetics.

(4) https://www.health.com/mind-body/healthy-immune-system-tips#:~:text=Manage%20your%20weight:%20Obesity% 20may,complications%20if%20you%20get%20sick.

(5) https://www.healthline.com/health/chronic-inflammation#:~:text=What%20causes%20chronic%20i nflammation?,industrial%20chemicals%20or%20pollut ed%20air

(6) ncy/article/000821.htm

(7) https://www.mdanderson.org/cancerwise/what-are-free-radicals-a-dietitian-explains.h00-159699912.html

(8) https://www.manhattangastroenterology.com/10-signs-you-may-have-a-parasite/#:~:text=Chronic%20Fatigue%20or%20Exhaust ion.%20Parasites%20are%20tough,and%20memory%2 0issues%20with%20feelings%20of%20apathy.

(9) https://sbiosd.com/drink-up-how-dehydration-fuels-back-pain/

(10) Unique lipoprotein phenotype and genotype associated with exceptional longevity - PubMed